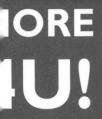

theclinics.com

This Clinics series is available online.

e's what
 get:

- Full text of EVERY issue from 2002 to NOW
- Figures, tables, drawings, references and more
- Searchable: find what you need fast

Search | All Clinics ▼ | for [ ] GO

- Linked to MEDLINE and Elsevier journals
- E-alerts

)IVIDUAL
BSCRIBERS

LOG ON TODAY. IT'S FAST AND EASY.

:k **Register**
 follow
tructions

 u'll need your
 ount number

Your subscriber
account number —
is on your mailing
label

This is your copy of:

THE CLINICS OF NORTH AMERICA

CXXX   **2296532-2**   2   Mar 05

J.H. DOE, MD
531 MAIN STREET
CENTER CITY, NY 10001-001

BOUGHT A SINGLE ISSUE? Sorry, you won't be able
to access full text online. Please subscribe today to get
complete content by contacting customer service at
800 645 2452 (US and Cana   ?45 4000 (outside
US and Canada) or via ema

D1154226

NEW!

Now also availab   S

ELSEVIER

Works/Integrates with MD Consult
Available in a variety of packages: Collections containing
14, 31 or 50 Clinics titles
Or Collection upgrade for existing MD Consult customers

Call today! 877-857-1047 or e-mail: mdc.groupinfo@elsevier.com

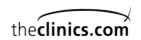

SURGICAL CLINICS
OF NORTH AMERICA

Bariatric Surgery

GUEST EDITOR
Edward H. Livingston, MD

CONSULTING EDITOR
Ronald F. Martin, MD

August 2005 • Volume 85 • Number 4

SAUNDERS

An Imprint of Elsevier, Inc.
PHILADELPHIA   LONDON   TORONTO   MONTREAL   SYDNEY   TOKYO

W.B. SAUNDERS COMPANY
A Division of Elsevier Inc.

1600 John F. Kennedy Blvd., Suite 1800, Philadelphia, PA 19103-2899

http://www.theclinics.com

SURGICAL CLINICS OF NORTH AMERICA
August 2005
Volume 85, Number 4
Editor: Catherine Bewick
ISSN 0039-6109
ISBN 1-4160-2793-9

Reprints. For copies of 100 or more of articles in this publication, please contact the commercial Reprints Department Elsevier Inc., 360 Park Avenue South, New York, New York 10010-1710. Tel. (212) 633-3813, Fax: (212) 462-1935, email: reprints@elsevier.com

The ideas and opinions expressed in *The Surgical Clinics of North America* do not necessarily reflect those of the Publisher. The Publisher does not assume any responsibility for any injury and/or damage to persons or property arising out of or related to any use of the material contained in this periodical. The reader is advised to check the appropriate medical literature and the product information currently provided by the manufacturer of each drug to be administered to verify the dosage, the method and duration of administration, or contraindications. It is the responsibility of the treating physician or other health care professional, relying on independent experience and knowledge of the patient, to determine drug dosages and the best treatment for the patient. Mention of any product in this issue should not be construed as endorsement by the contributors, editors, or the Publisher of the product or manufacturers' claims.

Surgical Clinics of North America (ISSN 0039-6109) is published bimonthly by Elsevier; Corporate and editorial Offices: 1600 John F. Kennedy Blvd., Suite 1800, Philadelphia, PA 19103-2899. Accounting and circulation offices: 6277 Sea Harbor Drive, Orlando, FL 32887-4800. Periodicals postage paid at Orlando, FL 32862, and additional mailing offices. Subscription prices are $190.00 per year for US individuals, $299.00 per year for US institutions, $95.00 per year for US students and residents, $234.00 per year for Canadian individuals, $365.00 per year for Canadian institutions, $250.00 for international individuals, $365.00 for international institutions and $125.00 per year for Canadian and foreign students/residents. To receive student/resident rate, orders must be accompanied by name of affiliated institution, date of term, and the *signature* of program/residency coordinator on institution letterhead. Orders will be billed at individual rate until proof of status is received. Foreign air speed delivery is included in all *Clinics* subscription prices. All prices are subject to change without notice. POSTMASTER: Send address changes to *The Surgical Clinics of North America*, W.B. Saunders Company, Periodicals Fulfillment, Orlando, FL 32887-4800. **Customer Service: 1-800-654-2452 (US). From outside of the US, call 1-407-345-1000.**

The Surgical Clinics of North America is also published in Spanish by McGraw-Hill Interamericana Editores S.A., P.O. Box 5-237 06500 Mexico D.F. Mexico; and in Portuguese by Interlivros Edicoes Ltda., Rua Comandante Coelho 1085, CEP 21250, Rio de Janeiro, Brazil; and in Greek by Paschalidis Medical Publications, Athens Greece.

The Surgical Clinics of North America is covered in *Index Medicus, EMBASE/Excerpta Medica, Current Contents/Clinical Medicine, Current Contents/Life Sciences, Science Citation Index*, and *ISI/BIOMED*.

Printed in the United States of America.

CONSULTING EDITOR

RONALD F. MARTIN, MD, Department of Surgery, Marshfield Clinic, Marshfield, Wisconsin; Clinical Associate Professor of Surgery, University of Vermont Medical College, Burlington, Vermont

GUEST EDITOR

EDWARD H. LIVINGSTON, MD, FACS, Hudsen-Penn Chair of Surgery, Professor and Chairman, Division of Gastrointestinal and Endocrine Surgery, University of Texas Southwestern School of Medicine, Dallas, Texas; Staff Surgeon, Veterans Administration, North Texas Health Care System, Dallas, Texas

CONTRIBUTORS

MOHAMED R. ALI, MD, Assistant Professor of Surgery, Department of Surgery; Director of Minimally Invasive/Bariatric Surgery, University of California Davis Medical Center, Sacramento, California

GARY J. ANTHONE, MD, FACS, Bariatric Surgery Program, Physicians Clinic, Nebraska Methodist Health System, Omaha, Nebraska

SUSAN BOWERMAN, MS, RD, Assistant Director, University of California Los Angeles Center for Human Nutrition, Los Angeles, California

ROBERT E. BROLIN, MD, Adjunct Professor of Surgery, University of Pittsburgh Medical Center, Pittsburgh, Pennsylvania; Director of Bariatric Surgery, University Medical Center at Princeton, Monmouth Junction, New Jersey

MICHAEL P. CHOI, DO, Fellow in Minimally Invasive Surgery, Department of Surgery, University of California Davis Medical Center, Sacramento, California

ERIC J. DeMARIA, MD, Chairman, Division of General Surgery and Director of Center for Minimally Invasive Surgery and the Obesity Surgery Program, Virginia Commonwealth University/Medical College of Virginia, Richmond, Virginia

WILLIAM D. FULLER, MD, Fellow in Minimally Invasive Surgery, Department of Surgery, University of California Davis Medical Center, Sacramento, California

WILLIAM G. HAYNES, MBChB, MD, Program Director and Professor, General Clinical Research Center, Carver College of Medicine, University of Iowa, Iowa City, Iowa

DAVID HEBER, MD, PhD, Professor of Medicine and Public Health, David Geffen School of Medicine at University of California Los Angeles; Director, University of California Los Angeles Center for Human Nutrition, Los Angeles, California

DONNA HEMINGWAY, MS, RD, Research Nutritionist, General Clinical Research Center, Carver College of Medicine, University of Iowa, Iowa City, Iowa

MOHAMMAD K. JAMAL, MD, Fellow, Division of General Surgery, Department of Surgery, Center for Minimally Invasive Surgery and the Obesity Surgery Program, Virginia Commonwealth University/Medical College of Virginia, Richmond, Virginia

JOHN G. KRAL, MD, PhD, Professor of Surgery and Medicine, Department of Surgery, State University of New York Downstate Medical Center, Brooklyn, New York

ZHAOPING LI, MD, PhD, Associate Clinical Professor of Medicine, David Geffen School of Medicine at University of California Los Angeles, Los Angeles, California

EDWARD H. LIVINGSTON, MD, FACS, Hudsen-Penn Chair of Surgery, Professor and Chairman, Division of Gastrointestinal and Endocrine Surgery, University of Texas Southwestern School of Medicine, Dallas, Texas; Staff Surgeon, Veterans Administration, North Texas Health Care System, Dallas, Texas

ERIK NÄSLUND, MD, PhD, Professor of Surgery, Division of Surgery, Karolinska Institute, Danderyd Hospital, Stockholm, Sweden

WALTER J. PORIES, MD, Professor of Surgery, Division of Bariatric Surgery, Brody School of Medicine at East Carolina University, Greenville, North Carolina

DAVID A. PROVOST, MD, Associate Professor of Surgery, Division of Gastrointestinal and Endocrine Surgery, Department of Surgery, The University of Texas Southwestern Medical Center at Dallas, Dallas, Texas; Director, Clinical Center for the Surgical Management of Obesity, the University of Texas Southwestern Medical Center at Dallas, Dallas, Texas

NANCY PUZZIFERRI, MD, Assistant Professor of Surgery, University of Texas Southwestern School of Medicine; Staff Surgeon, Veterans Administration North Texas Health Care System, Dallas, Texas

STEWART E. RENDON, MD, Clinical Assistant Professor of Surgery, Division of Bariatric Surgery, Brody School of Medicine at East Carolina University, Greenville, North Carolina

BASSEM Y. SAFADI, MD, FACS, Assistant Professor of Surgery, Stanford University; Staff Surgeon, Veterans Administration Palo Alto Health Care System, Palo Alto, California

PHYLLIS STUMBO, PhD, RD, Research Nutritionist, General Clinical Research Center, Carver College of Medicine, University of Iowa, Iowa City, Iowa

BRUCE M. WOLFE, MD, Professor Emeritus of Surgery, Department of Surgery, University of California Davis Medical Center, Sacramento, California

CONTENTS

undertaking with a special form of consumer product and service. In this day of limited resources and significant value exchanges among stakeholders (ie, patients, surgeons, third-party payers), the goal of the bariatric community is to deliver quality outcomes with safety, efficacy, and efficiency. The American Society for Bariatric Surgery and the Surgical Review Corporation, in conjunction with the bariatric community, will use quality assurance methods to produce quality outcomes that will satisfy the value exchanges of all stakeholders.

FORTHCOMING ISSUES

RECENT ISSUES

SURGICAL
CLINICS OF
NORTH AMERICA

ELSEVIER
SAUNDERS

Surg Clin N Am 85 (2005) xi–xii

Foreword

Bariatric Surgery

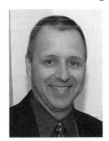

Ronald F. Martin, MD
Consulting Editor

It is ironic that with hunger being as prevalent in the world as it is that we should need to dedicate an issue of the *Surgical Clinics of North America* to the complication of excess caloric intake. Yet we do. During my career, I have seen few operations that have met with as much "dissention among the ranks" as bariatric procedures. Arguments have been made about the type of operation; on whom, by whom, and where they should be performed; and whether these procedures should be performed at all. Over the last few years, the use of these operations has increased in frequency dramatically. Some of this is clearly due to the increased ability to obtain third-party reimbursement, some is due to increased public awareness of the availability of bariatric procedures through celebrity patients, and some is secondary to the increase in potential candidates for these operations as the mean body mass index of our national population increases.

Many surgeons see operative intervention in the morbidly obese patient as a service to the "last systematically discriminated upon group," whereas others view it as the health care system compensating for lack of personal responsibility. There may be merit to either stance. However, if we collectively agreed to not treat people who have had some hand in their own medical problems, we would to a large extent discontinue health care— at least discontinue all care for diseases related to excess smoking, excess vehicular speed, and excess alcohol consumption, to name a few.

Dr. Livingston and his colleagues have collectively reviewed many of the issues that are central to the current discussion. Their thorough coverage of the topic will give those who favor as well as those who do not favor these

doi:10.1016/j.suc.2005.06.001   *surgical.theclinics.com*

procedures at least a common point of reference from which to continue the discussion.

With the current medico-economic climate as it is, it would seem likely that we as physicians and surgeons will have to get more serious about not just our individual responsibilities to our patients but also our collective responsibilities to the larger population from which our patients are derived. Many of the systems and economic issues that are brought up in the debates over bariatric surgery are representative of the larger, if you'll pardon the pun, patient problem in general; what costs can society bear for the few and how do we define and maintain quality medical care in a free market economy. Society, government, industry and our patients have all made it clear that they expect better health care for less money. Sadly, no one has defined what would constitute better, how much better do they want it to be or whom specifically it should be better for. Also, no one has been all that clear about how much (or little) individuals or society as a whole should be willing to pay for what is considered "better" health care.

In my opinion, waiting for politicians or agencies to resolve these questions for us is unlikely to work. It is with that in mind that I recommend reading the opinions and data put forth in this issue. Furthermore, as we continue in our efforts to make the *Surgical Clinics of North America* reflective of what each surgeon needs to know to practice effectively, I welcome your comments on this issue, as well as any other thoughts on what we can do to make this series important and relevant to the readership.

Ronald F. Martin, MD
Department of Surgery
Marshfield Clinic
1000 North Oak Avenue
Marshfield, WI 54449, USA

E-mail address: martin.ronald@marshfieldclinic.org

SURGICAL
CLINICS OF
NORTH AMERICA

ELSEVIER
SAUNDERS

Surg Clin N Am 85 (2005) xiii–xvii

Preface

Bariatric Surgery

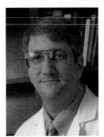

Edward H. Livingston, MD
Guest Editor

Obesity is increasing in epidemic proportions worldwide. Because obesity causes a variety of medical disorders, including hypertension and diabetes, it is feared that it will replace smoking as the most important reversible cause of reduced longevity. As a consequence, most public health agencies have recommended maintenance of a healthy weight and vigorous obesity treatment. Unfortunately, most obesity therapies have only minimal ability to induce sustained weight loss or comorbidity control. The exception is bariatric surgery. Consequently, the number of bariatric procedures performed in the United States has been increasing exponentially. Irrespective of the ability of various operations to induce long-term weight reduction and comorbidity control, surgical treatment of obesity has not been uniformly accepted by insurers or referring physicians. Because of the intense interest in bariatric surgery, this edition of *Surgical Clinics of North America* updates the current status of bariatric surgery.

The surge in obesity surgery has caused some insurance companies to limit coverage. Others have backed out of the obesity surgery market altogether. Many of those remaining have imposed restrictions that oftentimes appear arbitrary. Consequently, there has been a confusing array of major systematic reviews of bariatric surgery outcomes, with a variety of sometimes conflicting recommendations. Bassem Y. Safadi, MD, of Stanford University in Stanford, California, has summarized these in his article "Trends in Insurance Coverage for Bariatric Surgery and the Impact of Evidence-Based Reviews." In his summary, Dr. Safadi reviews recent changes that several major insurers have made in regards to limiting coverage for bariatric procedures. He also has compiled the finding of several of the recent major evidence-based reviews as they pertain to weight loss operations.

The basis for recommending weight loss surgery arises from the adverse health effects of obesity. Zaoping Li, MD, PhD, Susan Bowerman, MS, RD, and David Heber, MD, PhD, from the University of California Los Angeles (UCLA) Center for Human Nutrition provide a synopsis of the obesity epidemic and its consequences in their contribution entitled "Health Ramifications of the Obesity Epidemic." Virtually all authoritative bodies that have issued recommendations regarding obesity surgery state that nonsurgical means directed at weight loss should be attempted before bariatric procedures are offered. Phyllis Stumbo, PhD, RD, Donna Hemingway, MS, RD, and William G. Haynes, MB, ChB, MD, from the General Clinical Research Center of the University of Iowa's Carver College of Medicine in Iowa City, review the medical and pharmacological treatments of obesity in their article "Dietary and Medical Therapy of Obesity." Aside from reviewing obesity treatment in general, Dr. Stumbo and her colleagues provide recommendations for the management of postoperative bariatric surgery patients. Little has been written about how to manage these patients following their operations; thus this article provides important guidance for clinicians having this responsibility.

A fundamental difference between bariatric and other types of surgery is that weight loss operations impact not a structural, but rather a behavioral problem. Additionally, despite the great heterogeneity of body sizes, medical complications, and personality traits of patients undergoing these operations, most surgeons offer the same procedure type to all patients. Erik Näslund, MD, PhD, Professor of Surgery at the Karolinska Institutet in Stockholm, Sweden, and John Krall, MD, PhD, Professor of Surgery and Medicine at State University of New York Downstate Medical Center in Brooklyn, New York, address these matters in "Patient Selection and the Physiology of Gastrointestinal Antiobesity Operations." They provide a comprehensive review of the indications for the various operations. They have also reviewed the scientific underpinnings relied upon by major authoritative bodies that have issued obesity surgery guidelines. Drs. Naslund and Krall provide compelling arguments for the need to match individual patient's characteristics to a type of weight loss operation. This selection should be based on anticipated or desired outcomes. A detailed review of the physiological effects of bariatric procedures is also included.

As Drs. Naslund and Krall emphasize, bariatric procedures correct the manifestations of eating behaviors. Recognizing the linkage between psychology and obesity, many authoritative bodies and health insurers require mental health assessment before bariatric surgery. Despite this requirement, there has been a paucity of research in this area. What little is known about the relationship between psychology and bariatric surgery outcomes has been reviewed by Nancy Puzziferri, MD, from the University of Texas Southwestern School of Medicine Department of Surgery, in

Dallas, in her article "Psychological Issues in Bariatric Surgery—the Surgeon's Perspective." Unfortunately, preoperative psychological does not correlate with bariatric surgical outcomes. No single test exists that will predict a patient's response to surgery. Despite these limitations, Dr. Puzziferri provides guidance for the role of mental health providers in the care of perioperative bariatric patients, and highlights specific areas of research that should be pursued.

With the rise in bariatric procedures, there has been a perceived increase in complications and deaths from these elective operations. In spite of the fact that most bariatric surgical outcome studies have demonstrated morbidity and mortality rates equivalent to those of most other general surgical operations, malpractice litigation for weight loss operations remains a substantial problem. A large number of lawsuits and the public perception that there is a high mortality rate have harmed the reputation of weight loss operation, despite the successes these procedures have in inducing weight loss and controlling medical complications of obesity. In response to this problem, the American Society of Bariatric Surgery, led by Walter Pories, MD, has launched an initiative to develop Centers of Excellence for bariatric surgery. These Centers will meet certain minimum requirements for data gathering and reporting, and will have surgeons with substantial experience and facilities adequate to take care of overweight patients. The background and details of this process are reviewed in the article "Quality Assurance in Bariatric Surgery" by Stuart E. Rendon, MD and Walter J. Pories, MD, from the Division of Bariatric Surgery at the East Carolina University School of Medicine in Greenville, North Carolina.

Eric J. Demaria, MD and Mohammad K. Jamal, MD, from the Department of Surgery and Center for Minimally Invasive Surgery and Obesity Surgery Program at the Virginia Commonwealth University in Richmond, have summarized arguments against performing laparoscopic adjustable banding procedures. Their article is titled "Laparoscopic Adjustable Banding: Evolving Clinical Experience." They review arguments mitigating against performing these procedures. A discussion in favor of performing these procedures is provided in the article entitled "Laparoscopic Adjustable Gastric Banding: An Attractive Option" by David A. Provost, MD, from the Division of Gastrointestinal/Endocrine Surgery at the University of Texas Southwestern Medical Center. Dr. Provost has considerable experience in laparoscopic bariatric procedures and has accrued a large series of patients undergoing laparoscopic adjustable banding procedures. Based on his own personal outcomes and a summary of the literature, he argues in favor of broader application of laparoscopic banding procedures.

Several newer procedures have great promise for inducing weight loss in very large patients. The long-limb gastric bypass has been described by Robert E. Brolin, MD, Director of Bariatric Surgery at the University Medical Center in Princeton, New Jersey. Dr. Brolin is one of the pioneers in bariatric surgery, and he describes these procedures, which result in appreciable amounts of weight loss in superobese patients. A number of reports have demonstrated that these procedures are safe and induce acceptable levels of weight loss for patients otherwise refractory to gastric bypass procedures. Another operation, the duodenal switch procedure, avoids some of the complications of gastric bypass operations by leaving the gastric antrum in place. Iron deficiency anemia, one of the most difficult complications to manage following gastric bypass, is eliminated. The patients also do not suffer from "dumping syndrome," because the pylorus is intact, yet they experience considerable amounts of weight loss from this procedure. Gary J. Anthone, MD, from the bariatric surgical program of the Physicians Clinic in Nebraska Methodist Health System in Omaha, has contributed an article titled "The Duodenal Switch Operation for Morbid Obesity." Dr. Anthone has been performing this operation for many years and has achieved good outcomes.

The long-term results of bariatric procedures are for the most part good, but skeptics maintain that long-term complication rates are high and that medical comorbidity control is less than optimal. The status of current knowledge of long-term outcomes from these operations is summarized in an article entitled "Bariatric Surgical Outcomes," contributed by Mohammed R. Ali, MD, William D. Fuller, MD, Michael P. Choi, DO, and Bruce M. Wolfe, MD, from the University of California Davis Medical Center. Dr. Wolfe is the principal investigator of a multicenter, long-term National Institutes of Health (NIH) study examining the outcomes from these procedures. Although the current literature supporting favorable outcomes from these operations is overall positive, the NIH study that Dr. Wolfe heads will provide definitive answers regarding bariatric surgical procedure outcomes.

Finally, complications do occur in approximately 10% of patients undergoing bariatric surgical operations. Some of these complications can have devastating effects on patients if not managed promptly and appropriately. I have written an article entitled "Complications of Bariatric Surgery" summarizing what these adverse outcomes are, and, most importantly, providing advice regarding their management to reduce the impact any complication has on a patient's long-term outcome from the procedure.

Public demand, coupled with the lack of efficacy of nonsurgical treatment of obesity, ensures that these procedures will be more frequently performed in the general population. As the field of bariatric surgery evolves, there is now greater understanding regarding the pathophysiology of obesity and its treatment, and outcomes from medical and surgical approaches to treatment are better defined. This collection of articles provides the reader with the most recent state of knowledge regarding bariatric surgery, composed by a series of authors with known expertise in the areas they have written about. There is no doubt that when appropriately performed, bariatric operations are the most gratifying procedures general surgeons can perform. Weight loss is dramatic, comorbidity control is substantial, and patient satisfaction greater than for any other general surgical operation. Although these operations should be performed by experienced, well-trained surgeons, the characteristics of facilities and surgeons that are most associated with good outcomes are not well-defined.

At the time of this writing, there is no drug on the horizon with any potential to be as effective as surgery in controlling obesity. For these reasons all physicians need to have some degree of awareness regarding bariatric surgical operations, not only to know when to refer patients for these operations but how to manage them postoperatively. This edition of *Surgical Clinics of North America* provides the clinician with the necessary information to make decisions regarding bariatric surgical referrals and management.

Edward H. Livingston, MD
Gastrointestinal and Endocrine Surgery
University of Texas Southwestern School of Medicine
5323 Harry Hines Boulevard
Dallas, TX 75390-9156, USA

E-mail address: Edward.Livingston@UTSouthwestern.edu

SURGICAL
CLINICS OF
NORTH AMERICA

ELSEVIER
SAUNDERS

Surg Clin N Am 85 (2005) 665–680

Trends in Insurance Coverage for Bariatric Surgery and the Impact of Evidence-Based Reviews

Bassem Y. Safadi, MD, FACS[a,b,*]

[a]Department of Surgery, Stanford University, 300 Pasteur Drive, H 3591,
Stanford, CA 94305, USA
[b]VA Palo Alto Health Care System, 3801 Miranda Avenue, 112G, Palo Alto, CA 94304, USA

The number of bariatric surgical procedures that is performed in the United States has increased dramatically over the past decade [1]. This growth has been fueled by several factors, including the prevalence of morbid obesity in our society, the incorporation of laparoscopy to bariatric procedures, and the popularization of surgical treatment of obesity by the public and the media. Obesity and physical inactivity have become two of the most pressing and fastest growing health perils that face the United States [2,3]. The Surgeon General, Centers for Disease Control (CDC), and Department of Health and Human Services (HHS) continue to alert the public and medical community and emphasize the need for prevention and intervention, particularly in the young population [4,5]. Responding to calls from Secretary of HHS Tommy Thompson and the CDC, the Center for Medicare and Medicaid services (CMS) announced in October 2004 that the statement in the National Coverage Determinations Manual which stated that "obesity itself cannot be considered an illness" has been removed [6]. Not surprisingly, treatment options for obesity, including bariatric surgery, are receiving much more attention from various entities, including the public, medical community, interested government agencies, and third-party payers (TPPs).

Background

Historically, bariatric surgery has met with decades of skepticism and criticism, even within the surgical community itself. The concept of viewing

* VA Palo Alto Health Care System, 3801 Miranda Avenue, 112G, Palo Alto, CA 94304.
  E-mail address: bsafadi@stanford.edu

0039-6109/05/$ - Published by Elsevier Inc.
doi:10.1016/j.suc.2005.03.004
surgical.theclinics.com

obesity as a disease that should be treated took considerable time and effort to crystallize. The term "morbid obesity" was introduced by surgeon J. Howard Payne in the early 1960s to highlight that concept and convince insurance companies and other TPPs to reimburse the surgical treatment of obesity [7]. Efforts by Dr. Payne and many other pioneers in the field led to the evolution of bariatric surgery as we know it today. In 1991, those efforts culminated in the National Institutes of Health (NIH) consensus conference which outlined widely accepted guidelines and indications for the surgical treatment of morbid obesity. Those guidelines are still in effect today and are used by most bariatric surgeons in patient selection, work-up, and filing for insurance authorization. The 1991 conference concluded that there were sufficient data to recommend application of the Roux-en-Y gastric bypass (RYGB) or vertical band gastroplasty (VBG) for patients having a body mass index (BMI) of greater than 40 kg/m^2. The panel also recommended that surgery could be considered for patients with BMIs that ranged from 35 kg/m^2 to 40 kg/m^2 in the presence of serious obesity-related comorbidities. The panel acknowledged that limited data existed in support of these operations and recommended that further studies be performed to evaluate better the efficacy of surgical treatment of obesity. The NIH has not convened another conference, citing a lack of substantive new data that would change their earlier recommendations [8].

Since the 1991 conference, there have been few major changes in the field of bariatric surgery. Procedures, such as RYGB, bilio-pancreatic diversion (BPD), duodenal switch (DS), and gastric banding are now being performed by way of a minimal access approach [9]. These operations are technically demanding and require significant training and experience on the part of the surgeon. Laparoscopic RYGB, in particular, has been adopted widely and accounts for a large part of the recent growth in the number of bariatric procedures in the United States [10]. Laparoscopic adjustable gastric banding (LAGB) is the most common bariatric procedure that is performed outside the United States, and continues to gain wider acceptance in the United States [10,11]. The bariatric community is polarized over which procedure is the preferred method.

In the past decade, there has been an unprecedented increase in the number of bariatric procedures that are performed in the United States [1,10,12]. Media coverage of celebrities who have had weight loss surgery, such as Carnie Wilson and Al Roker, brought bariatric surgery closer to public awareness [13]. Medical claims related to bariatric surgery continue to increase and were predicted to exceed $5 billion in 2004 [14]. As a result, the TPPs were placed under significant pressure to reimburse these treatment modalities, and bariatric surgery is now under closer scrutiny. In addition to facing more claims for bariatric surgery, TPPs are now dealing with more surgeons and more hospitals that offer a variety of surgical approaches. The increase in demand for bariatric surgery has provided incentives, and in some cases, put pressures on some surgeons and hospitals to start weight loss surgical programs [14,15]. In some cases, this has resulted in bad outcomes when inexperienced surgeons and inadequately prepared facilities embarked upon these procedures. Bariatric surgical groups and individual surgeons do not have uniform standards of practice, and more importantly, have different outcomes, reporting, and charges for similar procedures. Leak rate, reoperation rate, and ICU stay, for example, may vary considerably between surgeons and between hospitals [1,9,12,16].

Insurance coverage trend

The changes in the field of bariatric surgery highlighted above led many TPP to either eliminate or reduce reimbursement for the surgical treatment of morbid obesity [14,17]. This undoubtedly impacted and will further impact a great number of patients, most of whom are unable to afford bariatric surgery without TPP coverage.

Restricting coverage

Most TPPs have restricted coverage of bariatric surgery (Table 1) [14,17]. Bariatric surgical practices today are experiencing an increase in preauthorization processing times and denials. Often, the letter of medical necessity requires documentation of patients' weights for periods of time that range from 1 to 5 years and documentation of failed dietary attempts at weight loss. Each plan's definition of dietary attempts varies, and in some cases, specifies that it be conducted with physician supervision for periods of time that range from 3 to 36 months. Arguably, these are legitimate screening tools, but, in effect, they eliminate many potentially eligible patients who failed to obtain or maintain accurate medical records. Some plans (as well as surgical groups) mandate a 5% to 10% weight loss before authorizing bariatric surgery. This strategy, in all likelihood, selects the motivated and potentially better candidates for surgery. Its use, however, has not been justified based on evidence [18]. Preoperative evaluation by a dietitian and psychologist is required almost universally but is not covered by some insurance plans. This, in turn, imposes a financial burden that some patients cannot afford. Many of these preoperative measures increase the time that it takes to become an eligible patient. Frequently, patients drop out because of frustration or because their insurance plans change. Although most denials that are based on medical necessity and failure to achieve eligibility criteria can be overturned eventually, many patients and physicians choose not to proceed with the appeals process [17].

Some TPPs have excluded certain procedures from coverage. Most reimburse open and laparoscopic RYGB, but many do not cover the LAGB or malabsorptive procedures, such as long-limb RYGB (LLRYGB), BPD, and DS. Aetna, for example, covers the LAGB only in certain conditions, such as cirrhosis of the liver, inflammatory bowel disease, extensive adhesions or history of multiple abdominal operations, and poorly controlled systemic disease (http://www.aetna.com/cpb/data/CPBA0157.html).

Table 1
Strategies adopted by some third-party payers to restrict coverage for bariatric surgery

Approach	Example
Eliminate coverage all together	BCBS Florida
Cover only certain procedures	Most cover RYGB, lap and open. Many do not cover LAGB, DS, mini-gastric bypass, gastric pacing
Restrict patient selection	Restrict age limits
	Guidelines other than NIH 1991 consensus conference (eg, BMI $> 50 kg/m^2$).
	Exclude patients based on risk profile
Create more obstacles for attaining eligibility	Lengthy preapproval process
	Letter of medical necessity:
	Definition and documentation of obesity duration
	Definition and documentation of dietary attempts at weight loss
	Mandatory 5–10% preoperative weight loss
	Preoperative work-up expense not covered
Restrict bariatric surgical centers/practices	ASBS Centers of Excellence (COE)
	BCBS COE of California/Wellpoint
	Health America and Health Assurance COE
	Kaiser Permanente
	The New York State Health Plans Association Bariatric project
Mandatory employment period before eligibility	1–3 years
Decrease or cap reimbursement	BCBS Michigan $10,000 lifetime cap for all treatment of obesity
Increase copay/deductible	

Abbreviations: ASBS, American Society for Bariatric Surgery; lap, laparoscopic.

Other approaches that TPPs have been adopting increasingly include decreasing physician and hospital payment. This may force many bariatric practices to close in today's environment of escalating malpractice premiums [19]. Another emerging trend is to shift more of the costs to patients and employers by increasing the deductible or by demanding a rider to secure coverage for bariatric surgery [14,20].

TPPs are aware that bariatric surgical outcomes differ from one practice to the other and also are aware that the costs of treating surgical complications is far greater than the cost of the primary procedure [14]. There is compelling evidence that mortality and complication rates decrease when there is a dedicated high-volume surgical group operating within a multidisciplinary team in a hospital with good resources [12,21,22]. This has led some insurance companies, employers, and hospital groups to designate centers of excellence (COE) to foster quality and control cost. Blue Cross Blue Shield (BCBS) of California/Wellpoint, for example, has been developing its own COE designation. The American Society for Bariatric Surgery has been proactive in developing and disseminating the COE concept through the Surgical

Review Corporation (http://www.surgicalreview.org/). This concept is in evolution at this stage, but undoubtedly will be the model that shapes bariatric surgical practices in the next few years.

Excluding coverage

The most dramatic and highly publicized event this year (2004) was the decision by BCBS of Florida (BCBSF) and Health Options, Inc. (HOI) to stop covering weight-loss surgeries as of January 2005 (http://www.bcbsfl.com). BCBSF/HOI stated that it "is choosing to join other health plans in excluding coverage for weight loss surgeries and services to protect the safety of our members and maintain the affordability of our products". Other large insurance carriers, such as Cigna, have excluded bariatric surgery under most of its plans (http://www.cigna.com/). When a TPP excludes coverage of any established therapeutic procedure, it gains some legal immunity [17]. If a given procedure is excluded entirely, the process of determining medical necessity becomes irrelevant, as does any subsequent external review process. There are other factors that influence the decision by TPPs to cover or exclude a given benefit, such as state legislation and insurance laws. Certain states, such as Georgia, Indiana, Maryland, and Virginia, have laws that require health plans to offer employers minimum coverage for morbid-obesity treatments, including bariatric surgery. These laws have limitations and can be challenged in court [17].

The employer also plays a vital role in determining whether to include bariatric surgery in its employees' health plan. This is particularly true for self-insured employers, which typically are large companies. These large companies frequently use TPPs to pay and administer their employees' benefits but ultimately assume the financial risk. As such, they have more leverage in shaping their employees' insurance plans and deciding which procedures to cover or exclude. For some employers who benefit from re-taining qualified employees long-term, bariatric surgery would pay off. It would help to retain healthier, more productive, and probably more satisfied employees. Studies from Quebec, Canada suggest that the cost of bariatric surgery may be recovered at approximately 3.5 years [23]. Conversely, employers with a high rate of turnover will be dissuaded by the increased up-front cost of bariatric surgery and may not be interested in covering it. A report by Mercer Human Resources Consulting this year revealed that only half of large companies that were surveyed had health plans that covered bariatric surgery (http://www.mercerhr.com/).

Medicare and bariatric surgery

The CMS is the largest payer entity in the United States and its coverage policies have tremendous effect on other TPPs which tend to follow CMS's position on most procedures and treatment modalities [20]. The recent change in the National Coverage Determinations (NCD) language did not change Medicare coverage policy on bariatric surgery [6]. Medicare has been covering bariatric surgery for at least 25 years. The indications for surgical treatment as stated in the NCD manual are not based on BMI, in contrast to the guidelines that were set by the 1991 NIH conference. Rather, the manual in section 40.5 states that "Gastric bypass surgery for extreme obesity is covered under the program if (1) it is medically appropriate for the individual to have such surgery; and (2) the surgery is to correct an illness which caused the obesity or was aggravated by the obesity (effective 10/1/1979)". The CMS is looking more closely at the role of bariatric surgery among Medicare beneficiaries (ie, mostly > 65 years old) and its role in patients who have obesity in the absence of serious morbidities. This prompted the Medicare Coverage Advisory Committee to conduct an evidence-based review on bariatric surgery, which was published in November of 2004 [24]. The review summary stated that "in general, there is evidence that weight loss is much higher in those patients with obesity who have bariatric surgery as compared with controls who do not have surgery" and that "bariatric surgery appears to have a place in the medical armamentarium of physicians treating obesity in the general population." It also acknowledged the beneficial effect of bariatric surgery on ameliorating obesity-related comorbidities and reducing years of life lost. Laparoscopic procedures were noted to have a lower complication rate than their counterpart open procedures, in general. It emphasized the role of surgeon experience in decreasing overall operative mortality and morbidity rates. The report concluded by pointing out that there is little scientific data on the efficacy and safety of bariatric surgery in patients older than 65 and cautioned that the available data do not allow generalization to the Medicare population.

Most bariatric practices set age limits (18 to 60 or 65 years) for determining eligibility, thereby excluding most Medicare patients (except for younger, but disabled patients who are on Medicare). Therefore, a change of coverage policy by Medicare will have little impact on practice referrals but will have a larger impact on how other TPPs cover bariatric surgery.

Evidence-based reviews

Periodically, the surgical treatment of obesity becomes a subject of a systematic review (Table 2). These often are referred to as evidence-based reviews or technology assessments and are sponsored or commissioned by a variety of sources, including government agencies, industry, hospital groups, or individual surgeons [16,24–28]. These reviews have significant impact on policy and often are quoted by TPPs to back certain claims which are related to weight loss surgery. Some of the reviews have significant flaws; a sample was chosen to highlight some of their limitations.

The Cochrane Review

The Cochrane Collaboration, founded in 1993, is an international nonprofit organization that produces and disseminates systematic reviews

Table 2
Examples of recent evidence-based reviews on bariatric surgery

Title [ref]	Source/year
A systematic review of laparoscopic adjustable gastric banding in the treatment of obesity	Australian Safety and Efficacy Register of New Interventional Procedures - Surgical (ASERNIP-S) 2000 (ASERNIP-S Report number 9).
Laparoscopic adjustable gastric banding for clinically severe (morbid) obesity	Schneider WL. Alberta Heritage Foundation for Medical Research 2000 (HTA 23):33.
Surgery for morbid obesity in adults	L'Agence Nationale d'Accreditation d'Evaluation en Sante 2001:4.
The clinical effectiveness and cost-effectiveness of surgery for people with morbid obesity: a systematic review and economic evaluation [26]	Clegg AJ, et al. The National Coordinating Centre for Health Technology Assessment on behalf of Southampton Health Technology Assessments Centre Southampton. 2002:153.
Surgery for morbid obesity [25]	Colquitt J, et al. Cochrane Database Syst Rev 2003;(2):CD003641
A systematic review of laparoscopic adjustable gastric banding for the treatment of obesity (update and re-appraisal)	Chapman A, et al. Australian Safety and Efficacy Register of New Interventional Procedures - Surgical (ASERNIP-S) 2002 (Report no 31):149.
Surgery for morbid obesity	Nilsen EM. Norwegian Health Services Research Centre 2003 (SMM-Report 1/2003).
Special report: the relationship between weight loss and changes in morbidity following bariatric surgery for morbid obesity	Blue Cross Blue Shield Association 2003 TEC Assesssment 18(9):1–25.
Newer techniques in bariatric surgery for morbid obesity [27]	Blue Cross Blue Shield Association 2003 TEC Assessment 18(10):1–51.
Laparoscopic adjustable gastric banding for morbid obesity.	Medical Services Advisory Committee (MSAC) 2003 (MSAC reference 14):153.
The gastric banding procedure: an evaluation	Chen J, McGregor M. Technology Assessment Unit of the McGill University Health Centre 2004:36.
Pharmacological and surgical treatment of obesity [16]	Shekelle PG, Morton SC, Maglione MA, et al. Agency for Healthcare Research and Quality 2004 (Evidence Report/Technology Assessment 103).
Summary of evidence—bariatric surgery	Brechner JR, Farries C, Harrison S, et al. Center for Medicaid Services. November 4, 2004
Bariatric surgery A systematic review and meta-analysis	Buchwald H, Avidor Y, Braunwald E, et al. JAMA 2004;292:1724–37.
Evidence-based medicine: open and laparoscopic bariatric surgery	Gentileschi P, Kini S, Catarci M, et al. Surg Endosc 2002;16(5):736–44.
Laparoscopic adjustable gastric banding in the treatment of obesity: a systematic literature review	Chapman AE, Kiroff G, Game P, et al. Surgery. 2004 Mar; 135(3):326–51.
Obesity surgery: evidence-based guidelines of the European Association for Endoscopic Surgery	Sauerland S, Angrisani L, Belachew M, et al. Surg Endosc 2005;19(2):200–21.

of health care interventions (http://www.cochrane.org/). Its major product is the Cochrane Database of Systematic Reviews which is published quarterly as part of The Cochrane Library. These publications are respected widely and often are quoted as evidence-based references [29]. The review on bariatric surgery was commissioned by the National Health Service Research and Development Health Technology Program (United Kingdom) on behalf of the National Institute of Clinical Excellence [25]. The stated objective was to assess the effects of bariatric surgery on weight, comorbidities, and quality of life. The review was published in 2004; the abstract can be found at http://www.cochrane.org//cochrane/revabstr/ab003641.htm. The investigators had published an earlier review in 2002 using similar methodology which reached essentially similar conclusions [26].

The Cochrane reviewers used strict methodology to extract references that were relevant to bariatric surgery. This is a common approach that is used in most evidence-based reviews or technology assessments. Reports queried for review were rated based on study methodology using criteria that were set by Jadad et al [30] and Schulz et al [31]. These criteria were developed to judge and rate the quality of randomized clinical trials (RCTs) and placed emphasis on factors, such as randomization, concealment of treatment allocation, and double-blinding. An RCT undoubtedly is the gold standard method for establishing "evidence-based surgery" and has been the model for validating procedures, such as breast-conserving resection for breast cancer and carotid endarterectomy for asymptomatic carotid artery disease [32,33]. RCTs rarely are conducted or reported for surgical procedures [29]. Most surgical results, including those of bariatric surgery, are reported in the form of case series and retrospective reviews which rank poorly in evidence grading. In the Cochrane review, 2608 (out of an original 2707) citations that were queried were excluded; 99 were retrieved for detailed examination. Only 18 trials reported in 33 publications were included; 17 were RCTs and 1 was a controlled clinical trial (CCT; Swedish Obese Subjects [SOS] trial). The most common reason for exclusion was study design other than an RCT or CCT. A total of 1891 patients formed the basis for the review (Table 3). Most of the patients were women between the ages of 33 and 47 years whose BMIs ranged from 41 kg/m^2 to 51 kg/m^2. The procedures included gastric bypass (34%), VBG (19%), horizontal gastroplasty (HGP) (18%) and gastric banding (9%). Malabsorptive procedures, such as DS and BPD, were not represented and only a small number of the procedures studied was laparoscopic [25].

Given the strict methodologic restrictions, the reviewers adopted a "tunnel vision" approach, rather than looking at the "big picture." Important contributions to the bariatric surgical literature, including large case series with long-term follow-up, were excluded [34–38]. Instead, emphasis was placed on trials that were fairly well-designed and conducted but have no clinical relevance today. One RCT, published in two reports in 1984 and 1988, compared surgical therapy with medical therapy for morbid

Table 3
The Cochrane Review. A summary of the trials selected for review

Treatment	Author	Year publication	N
Surgery versus conventional therapy	Andersen	1984/88	57
	SOS	1997–2000	483
GB versus VBG	Sugarman	1987	40
	VanWoert	1992	32
	Howard	1995	42
	MacLean	1995	106
GB versus VBG versus Band	Argen	1989	77
VBG versus HG	Laws	1981	53
	Lechner	1981	100
	Pories	1982	87
	Van Rij	1984	87
	Naslund	1988	57
GB versus HG versus VG	Hall	1990	310
VBG versus HG	Andersen	1987	45
VBG versus Band	Nilsell	2001	59
Open versus Lap GB	Nugyen	2001	155
	Westling	2001	51
Open versus Lap Band	DeWit	1999	50

Abbreviations: Band, gastric banding; GB, gastric bypass; HG, horizontal gastroplasty; VG, vertical gastroplasty.

obesity. The trial by Andersen et al [39,40] allocated 57 patients to a very low calorie diet (VLCD) or HGP, a procedure that is obsolete. In this trial, weight loss at 24 months was more pronounced in the surgical group (32 kg versus 9 kg; $P < 0.05$). At 5 years, success that was defined by a net weight loss of 10 kg was more common in the HGP group, although it did not represent a good outcome for a bariatric procedure (30% versus 17%). Results, such as the one published by Andersen et al, led to the abandonment of HGP and to the adoption of more durable procedures, such as the RYGB [8].

The other trial that was emphasized in this review is the SOS trial, a nonrandomized controlled clinical trial that compared patients who underwent surgery for morbid obesity with controls who were matched for 18 variables and followed prospectively [41–49]. The SOS trial reported a significantly ($P < 0.001$) greater weight loss at 2 years (23% versus 0%) and 5 years (16.3% versus 0.9% gain) in the surgical arm. Out of 251 surgical patients, 164 (65.3%) underwent VBG, a procedure that largely has been abandoned because of long-term failure. Only 24 patients (9.6%) underwent gastric bypass; they had a lower weight at 8 years than patients who had gastroplasty (P was not significant) or gastric banding ($P < 0.05$). In all likelihood, the weight loss at 5 years would have been more pronounced if all patients in the SOS trial had undergone a gastric bypass [16].

The reviewers reached the conclusion that "limited evidence suggests that surgery is more effective than conventional management for weight loss in morbid obesity. The comparative safety and effectiveness of different surgical procedures is unclear." The investigators continued by stating that "Good quality RCTs...comparing surgery with non-surgical treatment are needed." This proposition is not practical and arguably is unethical given the known effectiveness of surgical therapy and the poor results that generally are achieved with medical therapy [16,34,35,50].

The Blue Cross Blue Shield reviews

The technical assessment that was performed by the BCBS Technology Evaluation Center (TEC) in collaboration with Kaiser Permanente can be found at http://www.bcbs.com/tec/vol18/18_09.html [27]. The stated objective of the report was "to evaluate whether bariatric surgery improves health outcome for morbidly obese patients." The investigators used similarly restrictive selection criteria which yielded 18 reports of 13 studies. Six of the reports were from the SOS intervention trial, which was touted as the most important study in this review [45–49,51]. The Andersen et al [39,40] trial of VLCD versus HGP also was referenced. Eleven other single-arm reports were chosen. Those had data collected prospectively with a minimum follow-up of 1 year [52–62]. There was only one report on RYGB (79 patients) [54], three reports on VBG (222 patients) [58,60,61], three reports on gastric banding (159 patients) [55,56,59], two reports on BPD (93 patients) [52,53] and two reports on mixed surgery types (441 patients) [57,62]. The review concluded that "There is sufficient evidence to conclude that surgery improves health outcomes for patients with morbid obesity as compared with non surgical treatment. The best evidence is from the Swedish Obese Subjects (SOS) intervention trial, which has reported to date on several hundred patients in each group with up to 8 years of follow-up." The report continued to conclude, again based mostly on the SOS trial, that surgery improves quality of life and some comorbid conditions—diabetes, in particular. As in the Cochrane review, one of the major flaws with the BCBS evidence-based review was that rather than assess the sum total of the available literature, the investigators established criteria for the studies that they would evaluate. This resulted in a limited amount of data that the panels reviewed and upon which they based their conclusions.

Another highly publicized review by the BCBS TEC addressed the newer techniques in bariatric surgery, namely laparoscopic RYGB and laparoscopic gastric banding (LGB) in direct comparison with open RYGB [28]. In addition, the report focused on procedures that were not covered previously, such as BPD and LLRYGB. The report was published in September 2003; the abstract can be found at http://www.bcbs.com/tec/vol18/18_10.html. The review starts with a preface that "gastric bypass with Roux-en-Y anastomosis has been considered the bariatric surgery of choice in the United States, and this is supported by a substantial body of literature." The review also acknowledged that nonsurgical treatments have limited success in achieving substantial weight loss for morbidly obese patients. The literature selection criteria were not as restrictive in this review. Included were large case series from surgeons who pioneered the field of laparoscopic bariatric surgery, such as Higa et al [63] and Schauer et al [64]. Despite that, the reviewers concluded that there was insufficient evidence to recommend any laparoscopic bariatric procedure, BPD, or LLRYGB in the presence of current established surgery, namely open RYGB. The main reason for reaching this conclusion on laparoscopic RYGB was the rates of anastomotic leak (1%–6%) and obstruction (0%–10%) that were quoted in RCTs and single-arm studies. One of the RCTs that was published by Westling and Gustavsson [65] reported unusually high rates of operative mortality (3%), conversion (23%), and anastomotic complications (23%) in the laparoscopic arm (30 patients). Another comparative study by See et al [66] reported a series of 20 patients who underwent laparoscopic RYGB with 5% mortality and 20% incidence of anastomotic leaks. The number of patients in both series is small and the poor result undoubtedly is a reflection of the surgeons' inexperience with the laparoscopic approach. Laparoscopic RYGB is a technically difficult and challenging operation but several bariatric surgical groups have demonstrated that it can be performed safely and effectively [9,63,64,67]. These data should not be used to discard or discredit the operation but rather to define how and by whom it should be performed.

The main reasons that were cited for not supporting LGB were the poorer weight loss that was achieved at 1-year compared with open RYGB and a the rates of long-term adverse events, such as band erosion and slippage. The report acknowledged that LGB is technically less complex and is associated with fewer early adverse events compared with RYGB. It also pointed out that the difference in weight loss may lessen over time as evidenced by 3-year weight loss reports. The review did not take into account that LGB has been evolving over the past decade. Many of the problems, such as band erosion and slippage, are now understood better and have been reduced with changes in placement technique. In addition, newer designs have reduced the problems that are related to tube breakage and malfunction significantly. Intermediate follow-up in patients who underwent LGB suggest that in contrast to RYGB, weight loss continues beyond the first year [11,68,69]. Using 1-year weight as an outcome measure is not going to give justice to the band.

The so-called "evidence-based reviews" that were presented above reached conclusions that are not valid. The reviewers had a skewed interpretation of available data and did not evaluate procedures in the context of their evolution or in terms of their relevance today. Not surprisingly, these reviews were created without the participation of recognized experts in bariatric surgery. For the BCBS reviews, an inherent bias or conflict of interest may have played a role in shaping the reviews' conclusions. There is little doubt that laparoscopy makes bariatric surgery more appealing to patients. An industry-sponsored review is more likely to discourage procedures that would increase the demand for more coverage.

The RAND/Agency for Health Care Research and Quality review

A more comprehensive evidence-based review recently was completed by the RAND Corporation on contract with the Agency for Health Care Research and Quality [16]. This panel avoided the mistakes of the previously cited efforts by including a large consulting group of known experts in the field of bariatric surgery. These individuals worked in consultation with health care researchers who had specific expertise in the analysis of published literature and outcomes studies. The panel categorized and reviewed all of the available bariatric surgery literature (142 studies included in the final analysis). The review titled "Pharmacological and Surgical Treatment of Obesity" can be accessed at http://www.ncbi.nlm.nih.gov/books/bv.fcgi?rid=hstat1a.chapter.19289. The conclusions were that bariatric surgery is more effective than nonsurgical treatment and clearly results in sustained weight loss and comorbidity control for a group of patients with a BMI greater than 40 kg/m^2. For patients with a BMI between 35 kg/m^2 and 40 kg/m^2, the report stated that the data strongly support the superiority of surgical therapy but it cannot be considered conclusive. The review concluded that RYGB, VBG, and adjustable banding all result in sustained weight loss, but that RYGB is superior to VBG. Laparoscopic gastric bypass procedures have roughly equivalent outcomes to their open counterparts if well-trained, experienced surgeons perform them. The main advantage of laparoscopic procedures is the reduction of wound-related complications and incisional hernias.

Recommendations for future research by this group also was more reasonable; they stated that at this stage an RCT that compares medical and surgical therapies is not warranted given the known superiority of the latter. That might change should there be significant advances in nonsurgical therapy, or should eligibility criteria for bariatric surgery relax to include lower BMIs. Instead, the reviewers suggested obtaining data from well-conducted observational studies that are similar to the SOS trial, and looking for factors that might identify subgroups of patients for benefit/risk stratification. In addition, more RCTs were recommended for comparing the effectiveness and safety of different surgical procedures.

Summary

The demand for bariatric surgery is expected to continue to increase as long as there is no effective alternative for the treatment of morbid obesity. Surgery costs may be recovered in a few years, but the reality is that the up-front costs are high. Given the large number of potential patients, TPPs are facing increased pressure to reimburse these procedures. Some have responded proactively with patients and surgeons with a move to designate centers of excellence that provide the quality service at controlled cost. Others have responded by excluding or reducing coverage. The response is based on the notion that bariatric surgery or certain procedures are "unproven" or "experimental." Some evidence-based reviews with significant flaws often are cited to back those claims. These reviews generally conclude that the quality of outcomes research in bariatric surgery is poor. Such comments should be an impetus for bariatric surgeons to be more aggressive in leading prospective, high-quality trials and aim to standardize the technical aspects of each procedure.

References

[1] Pope GD, Birkmeyer JD, Finlayson SR. National trends in utilization and in-hospital outcomes of bariatric surgery. J Gastrointest Surg 2002;6:855–61.

[2] Flegal KM, Carroll MD, Kuczmarski RJ, et al. Overweight and obesity in the United States: prevalence and trends, 1960–1994. Int J Obes Relat Metab Disord 1998;22:39–47.

[3] Mokdad AH, Serdula MK, Dietz WH, et al. The spread of the obesity epidemic in the United States, 1991–1998. JAMA 1999;282:1519–22.

[4] McTigue KM, Harris R, Hemphill B, et al. Screening and interventions for obesity in adults: summary of the evidence for the US Preventive Services Task Force. Ann Intern Med 2003; 139(11):933–49.

[5] The Surgeon General's Call to Action to Prevent and Decrease Overweight and Obesity. Available at: http://www.surgeongeneral.gov/topics/obesity. Accessed March 10, 2005.

[6] CMS Manual System. Department of Health and Human Services Centers for Medicare and Medicaid Services. Pub. 100–03, Medicare National Coverage Determinations. Transmittal 23; October 1, 2004.

[7] Kral JG. Morbidity of severe obesity. Surg Clin North Am 2001;81(5):1039–61.

[8] Consensus Development Conference Panel. Gastrointestinal surgery for severe obesity. Ann Intern Med 1991;115:956–61.

[9] Cottam DR, Mattar SG, Schauer PR. Laparoscopic era of operations for morbid obesity. Arch Surg 2003;138(4):367–75.

[10] Buchwald H, Williams SE. Bariatric surgery worldwide 2003. Obes Surg 2004;14(9):1157–64.

[11] Ren CJ, Weiner M, Allen JW. Favorable early results of gastric banding for morbid obesity: the American experience. Surg Endosc 2004;18(3):543–6.

[12] Flum DR, Dellinger EP. Impact of gastric bypass operation on survival: a population-based analysis. J Am Coll Surg 2004;199(4):543–51.

[13] Johnson P. The skinny on Roker's weight loss: gastric bypass. USA Today. November 4, 2002; Life section, p. 3.

[14] Alt SJ. Bariatric surgery may become a self-pay service. Health Care Strateg Manage 2003; 21(12):12–9.

[15] Alt SJ. Bariatric surgery programs growing quickly nationwide. Health Care Strateg Manage 2001;19(9):7–23.

[16] Shekelle PG, Morton SC, Maglione MA, et al. Pharmacological and surgical treatment of obesity. Evidence Report/Technology Assessment No. 103. AHRQ Publication #04–E028–2. Rockville (MD): Agency for Healthcare Research and Quality; 2004.

[17] Hall MA. State regulation of medical necessity: the case of weight-reduction surgery. Duke Law J 2003;53(2):653–72.

[18] California Department of Managed Health Care. Review of weight loss prior to bariatric surgery. Available at: http://www.dmhc.ca.gov/boards/cap/BariatricREV.pdf. Accessed March 10, 2005.

[19] Baker JW. Excerpt from "Will a Surgeon be There." ASBS Newsletter Fall 2004;7–12.

[20] Fuhrmans V. Medicare mulls coverage shift on obesity as panel takes up issue of surgery for weight loss, private carriers begin covering more treatments. The Wall Street Journal. November 3, 2004; section D:1.

[21] Courcoulas A, Schuchert M, Gatti G, et al. The relationship of surgeon and hospital volume to outcome after gastric bypass surgery in Pennsylvania: a 3-year summary. Surgery 2003; 134:613–23.

[22] Nguyen NT, Paya M, Stevens CM, et al. The relationship between hospital volume and outcome in bariatric surgery at academic medical centers. Ann Surg 2004;240(4): 586–93.

[23] Sampalis JS, Liberman M, Auger S, et al. The impact of weight reduction surgery on health-care costs in morbidly obese patients. Obes Surg 2004;14(7):939–47.

[24] Brechner RJ, Farris C, Harrison S, et al. Summary of evidence—bariatric surgery. November 4, 2004. http://www.cms.hhs.gov/mcac/id137c.pdf. Accessed March 10, 2005.

[25] Colquitt J, Clegg A, Sidhu M. Surgery for morbid obesity (Cochrane review). In: The Cochrane Library. Chichester, UK: John Wiley and Sons, Ltd; 2004. p. 1–56.

[26] Clegg AJ, Colquitt J, Sidhu MK, et al. The clinical effectiveness and cost-effectiveness of surgery for people with morbid obesity: a systematic review and economic evaluation. Health Technol Assess 2002;6(12). p. 1–151.

[27] Blue Cross Blue Shield Association. Special report: the relationship between weight loss and changes in morbidity following bariatric surgery for morbid obesity. Technol Eval Center Asses Progr Exec Summ 2003;18(9):1–25.

[28] Blue Cross Blue Shield Association. Newer techniques in bariatric surgery for morbid obesity. Technol Eval Center Asses Progr Exec Summ 2003;18(10):1–51.

[29] Rikkers LF. The bandwagon effect. J Gastrointest Surg 2002;6(6):787–94.

[30] Jadad AR, Moore RA, Carroll D, et al. Assessing the quality of reports of randomized clinical trials: is blinding necessary? Control Clin Trials 1996;17(1):1–12.

[31] Schulz KF, Chalmers I, Hayes RJ, et al. Empirical evidence of bias. Dimensions of methodological quality associated with estimates of treatment effects in controlled trials. JAMA 1995;273(5):408–12.

[32] Fisher B, Anderson S, Redmond CK, et al. Reanalysis and results after 12 years of follow-up in a randomized clinical trial comparing total mastectomy with lumpectomy with or without irradiation in the treatment of breast cancer. N Engl J Med 1995;333(22):1456–61.

[33] Executive Committee for the Asymptomatic Carotid Atherosclerosis Study. Endarterectomy for asymptomatic carotid artery stenosis. JAMA 1995;273(18):1421–8.

[34] MacDonald KGJ, Long SD, Swanson MS, et al. The gastric bypass operation reduces the progression and mortality of non-insulin-dependent diabetes mellitus. J Gastrointest Surg 1997;1:213–20.

[35] Pories WJ, Swanson MS, MacDonald KG, et al. Who would have thought it? An operation proves to be the most effective therapy for adult-onset diabetes mellitus. Ann Surg 1995;222: 339–50.

[36] Hess DS, Hess DW. Biliopancreatic diversion with a duodenal switch. Obes Surg 1998;8: 267–82.

[37] Marceau P, Hould FS, Simard S, et al. Biliopancreatic diversion with duodenal switch. World J Surg 1998;22:947–54.

[38] Scopinaro N, Adami GF, Marinari GM, et al. Biliopancreatic diversion. World J Surg 1998; 22:936–46.

[39] Andersen T, Backer OG, Stokholm KH, et al. Randomized trial of diet and gastroplasty compared with diet al.one in morbid obesity. N Engl J Med 1984;310(6):352–6.

[40] Andersen T, Stokholm KH, Backer OG, et al. Long-term (5-year) results after either horizontal gastroplasty or very-low-calorie diet for morbid obesity. Int J Obes 1988;12(4): 277–84.

[41] Karason K, Lindroos AK, Stenlof K, et al. Relief of cardiorespiratory symptoms and increased physical activity after surgically induced weight loss: results from the Swedish Obese Subjects study. Arch Intern Med 2000;160(12):1797–802.

[42] Karason K, Molgaard H, Wikstrand J, et al. Heart rate variability in obesity and the effect of weight loss. Am J Cardiol 1999;83(8):1242–7.

[43] Karason K, Wallentin I, Larsson B, et al. Effects of obesity and weight loss on left ventricular mass and relative wall thickness: survey and intervention study. BMJ 1997;315(7113):912–6.

[44] Karason K, Wikstrand J, Sjostrom L, et al. Weight loss and progression of early atherosclerosis in the carotid artery: a four-year controlled study of obese subjects. Int J Obes Relat Metab Disord 1999;23(9):948–56.

[45] Karlsson J, Sjöström L, Sullivan M. Swedish obese subjects (SOS): an intervention study of obesity: two-year follow-up of health-related quality of life (HRQL) and eating behavior after gastric surgery for severe obesity. Int J Obes Relat Metab Disord 1998;22:113–26.

[46] Narbro K, Agren G, Jonsson E, et al. Sick leave and disability pension before and after treatment for obesity: a report from the Swedish Obese Subjects (SOS) study. Int J Obes Relat Metab Disord 1999;23(6):619–24.

[47] Sjostrom CD, Lissner L, Wedel H, et al. Reduction in incidence of diabetes, hypertension and lipid disturbances after intentional weight loss induced by bariatric surgery: the SOS Intervention Study. Obes Res 1999;7(5):477–84.

[48] Sjostrom CD, Peltonen M, Sjostrom L. Blood pressure and pulse pressure during long-term weight loss in the obese: the Swedish Obese Subjects (SOS) Intervention Study. Obes Res 2001;9(3):188–95.

[49] Sjostrom CD, Peltonen M, Wedel H, et al. Differentiated long-term effects of intentional weight loss on diabetes and hypertension. Hypertension 2000;36(1):20–5.

[50] Christou NV, Sampalis JS, Lieberman M, et al. Surgery decreases long-term mortality, morbidity, and health care use in morbidly obese patients. Ann Surg 2004;240:416–23.

[51] Agren G, Narbro K, Naslund I, et al. Long-term effects of weight loss on pharmaceutical costs in obese subjects. A report from the SOS intervention study. Int J Obes Relat Metab Disord 2002;26(2):184–92.

[52] Adami GF, Meneghelli A, Bressani A, et al. Body image in obese patients before and after stable weight reduction following bariatric surgery. J Psychosom Res 1999;46(3):275–81.

[53] Adami GF, Gandolfo P, Meneghelli A, et al. Binge eating in obesity: a longitudinal study following biliopancreatic diversion. Int J Eat Disord 1996;20(4):405–13.

[54] Choban PS, Onyejekwe J, Burge JC, et al. A health status assessment of the impact of weight loss following Roux-en-Y gastric bypass for clinically severe obesity. J Am Coll Surg 1999; 188(5):491–7.

[55] Dixon JB, O'Brien PE. Health outcomes of severely obese type 2 diabetic subjects 1 year after laparoscopic adjustable gastric banding. Diabetes Care 2002;25(2):358–63.

[56] Freys SM, Tigges H, Heimbucher J, et al. Quality of life following laparoscopic gastric banding in patients with morbid obesity. J Gastrointest Surg 2001;5(4):401–7.

[57] Hawke A, O'Brien P, Watts JM, et al. Psychosocial and physical activity changes after gastric restrictive procedures for morbid obesity. Aust N Z J Surg 1990;60(10):755–8.

[58] Kalfarentzos F, Kechagias I, Soulikia K, et al. Weight loss following vertical banded gastroplasty: intermediate results of a prospective study. Obes Surg 2001;11(3):265–70.

[59] Larsen F, Torgersen S. Personality changes after gastric banding surgery for morbid obesity. A prospective study. J Psychosom Res 1989;33(3):323–34.

[60] Melissas J, Christodoulakis M, Schoretsanitis G, et al. Obesity-associated disorders before and after weight reduction by vertical banded gastroplasty in morbidly vs super obese individuals. Obes Surg 2001;11(4):475–81.

[61] Melissas J, Christodoulakis M, Spyridakis M, et al. Disorders associated with clinically severe obesity: significant improvement after surgical weight reduction. South Med J 1998; 91(12):1143–8.

[62] Powers PS, Rosemurgy A, Boyd F, et al. Outcome of gastric restriction procedures: weight, psychiatric diagnoses, and satisfaction. Obes Surg 1997;7(6):471–7.

[63] Higa KD, Ho T, Boone KB. Laparoscopic Roux-en-Y gastric bypass: technique and 3-year follow-up. J Laparoendosc Adv Surg Tech 2001;11(6):377–82.

[64] Schauer PR, Ikramuddin S, Gourash W, et al. Outcomes after laparoscopic Roux-en-Y gastric bypass for morbid obesity. Ann Surg 2000;232(4):515–29.

[65] Westling A, Gustavsson S. Laparoscopic vs open Roux-en-Y gastric bypass: a prospective, randomized trial. Obes Surg 2001;11(3):284–92.

[66] See C, Carter PL, Elliott D, et al. An institutional experience with laparoscopic gastric bypass complications seen in the first year compared with open gastric bypass complications during the same period. Am J Surg 2002;183(5):533–8.

[67] Schauer P, Ikramuddin S, Hamad G, et al. The learning curve for laparoscopic Roux-en-Y gastric bypass is 100 cases. Surg Endosc 2003;17(2):212–5.

[68] Ren CJ. Controversies in bariatric surgery: evidence-based discussions on laparoscopic adjustable gastric banding. J Gastrointest Surg 2004;8(4):396–7.

[69] Fielding GA, Ren CJ. Laparoscopic adjustable gastric band. Surg Clin North Am 2005; 85(1):129–40.

ELSEVIER
SAUNDERS

SURGICAL
CLINICS OF
NORTH AMERICA

Surg Clin N Am 85 (2005) 681–701

Health Ramifications of the Obesity Epidemic

Zhaoping Li, MD, PhD[a],*, Susan Bowerman, MS, RD[b],
David Heber, MD, PhD[a,b]

[a]David Geffen School of Medicine at UCLA, 12-105 Center for Health Sciences,
Box 957035, Los Angeles, CA 90095-7035, USA
[b]UCLA Center for Human Nutrition, 900 Veteran Avenue, Los Angeles,
CA 90095-1742, USA

Obesity has been defined as excess body fat relative to lean body mass [1], and in humans is the result of interactions of the environment with multiple genes. Although humans are well adapted to starvation, they are poorly adapted to overnutrition. In fact, only for the past 100 years have humans had a continuous surplus of food. The modern high-fat, high-calorie diet combined with physical inactivity has resulted in an epidemic of obesity and overweight.

The age-adjusted prevalence of obesity was 30.5% in 1999 to 2000 [2]. Despite the fact that a precise estimate of the change in the prevalence of obesity over time is difficult because of changing definitions, nearly all clinical authorities agree that obesity is reaching epidemic proportions [2–10]. Although obesity is excess adiposity, a convenient parameter for documenting the incidence of obesity and for setting clinical guidelines is the body mass index (BMI), which is expressed as body weight (in kilograms) divided by the height (in meters) squared. Individuals whose BMI is greater than 30 are obese, whereas those whose BMI is between 25 and 29.9 are termed *overweight*. There are also further classifications of obesity, including severe obesity or class I, II, or III, based on BMI.

Prevalence of obesity

The increasing prevalence of overweight and obesity among American adults and children has been identified as an epidemic by the Surgeon General and as one of the Leading Health Indicators for Healthy People

---

* Corresponding author.
E-mail address: zli@mednet.ucla.edu (Z. Li).

2010 [11,12]. The prevalence of obesity has been increasing over the past 25 years, as defined in representative United States health examination surveys [8,9]. Between 1976 and 1994, the prevalence of obesity (defined as BMI $\geq$ 30 kg/m^2) among men and women aged 20 to 74 years rose sharply from 14.5% to 22.5%. During the same period, the prevalence of overweight and obesity combined (defined as BMI $\geq$ 25 kg/m^2) increased markedly from 32% to 55% [9].

The prevalence of women who are overweight or obese is even higher in nonwhite populations. Among the non-Hispanic black and Mexican-American respondents in the National Health and Nutrition Examination Survey (NHANES) III, 20% of the men and approximately 35% of the women were obese [13].

The United States is not alone in facing rising rates of obesity. In Canada, the prevalences of overweight and obesity have increased from 40.0% and 9.7% in 1970 to 1972 to 50.7% and 14.9% in 1998, respectively. The entire BMI distribution has shifted to the right since 1970 to 1972 and has become more skewed to the right for men than for women [14]. In a cohort study of children born in 1997, 25.6% of the preschool children were overweight or obese [15]. The World Health Organization (WHO) reports that there are more than 300 million obese people in the world, and the rising rate of obesity is no longer solely a problem of industrialized countries but is also rapidly appearing in developing countries [3,16].

It is less common to be overweight (BMI = 25–29.9) in most European countries than it is in the United States, but the prevalence of overweight adults in Germany, Finland, and Britain is more than 50%. Obesity (BMI $\geq$ 30) also is generally less common in Europe than in the United States, occurring in approximately 10% to 20% of adult men and 15% to 25% of women [17]. In Western European study centers participating in the WHO multinational monitoring of determinants and trends in cardiovascular disease (MONICA) study, the prevalence of obesity in individuals aged 35 to 64 years ranged from 10% to 24% among men and from 9% to 25% among women in 1989 to 1996. Obesity was more common in Eastern Europe, especially among women. In Polish and Russian study centers, the prevalence of obesity was around 40% [18].

The prevalence of obesity is not only increasing rapidly in industrialized countries but also in nonindustrialized countries, particularly those undergoing economic transition [19]. Worldwide, nearly 250 million people are obese, and the WHO has estimated that in 2025, 300 million people will be obese [20]. Attitudes toward obesity differ across populations and, with economic changes, may change within populations over time. In industrialized countries, obesity is most common among those who have low socioeconomic status, but the opposite is true in nonindustrialized countries where obesity is most often seen among individuals who have high incomes, and may be considered a status symbol. This may change as nonindustrialized countries become more affluent and obesity becomes more prevalent in individuals who have low socioeconomic status. Bell et al [21] studied a cohort of 2488 adults aged 20 to 45 years in 1989 drawn from seven provinces in China using multistage, random cluster sampling, with weight change over 8 years as the outcome variable. Overweight (BMI > 25) doubled in women (10.4%–20.8%) and almost tripled in men (5.0%–14.1%).

Obesity in children and adolescents

According to the most recent results of the NHANES, 15.5% of adolescents are currently overweight [14] and are displaying increasing rates of obesity-related chronic diseases not previously seen in children [6], such as type II diabetes mellitus (T2DM). The prevalence of overweight and obesity among children appears to be rising rapidly in many countries in Europe. Several European countries have made estimates of the prevalence of childhood overweight and obesity during the last decade. In a recent survey, the highest prevalence of overweight (85th percentile BMI of the studied population) in Europe among 13-year-olds is equally divided between countries representing different regions, such as Finland, Ireland, and Greece. In the same study, it is clear that the highest prevalence of overweight in Europe is approaching United States levels [22].

Children in China are also getting fatter [23]. In urban areas in China, the prevalence of childhood obesity increased from 1.5% in 1989 to 12.6% in 1997 and prevalence of overweight increased from 14.6% to 28.9% in the same period [24]. In a more recent study reported from China, the prevalence of overweight for children was 27.7% in boys and 14.1% in girls [25]. By the end of 2000, the obesity rate of male students in Beijing, China reached 15%, doubling that of 1990 and approaching that of developed countries, as indicated by the National Physique Survey in 2000, which was jointly launched by the State Sports General Administration, Ministry of Education, and nine other ministries and commissions [23].

Obesity and public health

The health consequences of obesity include some of the most common chronic diseases in our society. Obesity is an independent risk factor for heart disease [26], the most common killer disease in most developed countries. T2DM, hypertension, stroke, hyperlipidemia, osteoarthritis (OA), and sleep apnea are all more common in obese individuals. A recent prospective study involving 900,000 United States adults reported that increased body weight was associated with increased death rates for all cancers combined and for cancers at multiple specific sites [27]. Adult weight gain is associated with increased risk for breast cancer in postmenopausal women [28]. In the Diabetes Prevention Program, a weight loss of about 5% to 6% among persons with a BMI of 34 kg/m^2, along with increased physical activity, resulted in a 58% reduction in the incidence of diabetes [29].

Obesity and mortality

Recent studies have reaffirmed high BMI levels as risk factors for all-cause mortality [30,31]. Mortality risk increased for BMI above 27 kg/m^2 in the Nurses' Health Study [32] and the US Health Professionals Follow-Up Study [33].

In the recently published Physicians' Health Study [34], 85,078 men aged 40 to 84 years were followed for 5 years. In all age strata (40–54, 55–69, and 70–84 years), never-smokers who had BMIs of 30 or more had approximately a 70% increased risk for death compared with the referent group (BMI = 22.5–24.9). Higher levels of BMI were also strongly related to increased risk for cardiovascular mortality, regardless of physical activity level.

Calle and colleagues [35] concluded that the relation between high BMI and increased mortality was more pronounced in white than in black people and was stronger among never-smokers than among smokers. Their analysis was based on follow-up of more than 1 million United States men and women aged 30 years and over (mean age of 57 years) from 1982 through 1996.

These studies demonstrated a U-shaped relation between BMI and all-cause mortality in men and women. Lean men (BMI < 20) did not have excess mortality, regardless of age [34]. Lean women also did not have excess mortality. The lowest mortality rate was observed among women who weighed at least 15% less than the United States average for women of similar age and among those whose weight had been stable since early adulthood [32].

Obesity and diabetes

When one examines the risk for T2DM and BMI, the relationship is out of proportion to the relative risks for other obesity-related diseases and is in the range of a 60- to 80-fold increased risk at a BMI of 30 [36]. This is not a risk factor at 8000%, but evidence of an intrinsic interrelationship in terms of genetics, environment, and pathophysiology between obesity and T2DM, which has been termed "diabesity" [37]. Furthermore, there is evidence that obesity worsens the metabolic abnormalities often associated with T2DM, including hyperinsulinemia, hyperglycemia, hypertension, and hyperlipidemia. It has been estimated that more than 70% of all individuals who have T2DM are overweight and that one third are obese [38].

The WHO has predicted that the number of diabetics will double from 143 million in 1997 to about 300 million in 2025, largely because of dietary and other lifestyle factors [20]. It has been calculated that in whites, 65% to 75% of incident cases of diabetes could be avoided if the population as a whole did not exceed a BMI of 25 [39,40]. Adult weight gain, the degree of obesity, and the duration of obesity independently and strongly predict the risk for T2DM [41].

In Asian countries, the prevalence of T2DM will increase more rapidly over time than the increase in obesity [19]. There are many indications that the risk for diabetes starts to increase rapidly at BMI values or waist circumference measurements well in the acceptable range of BMI or waist circumference for Europeans [42]. This may imply that cut-off points, as recommended for white populations (BMI > 30, waist larger than 88 cm in women or 102 cm in men), have little value for identifying Asian individuals who are at high risk and who constitute more than half of the world's population. Lowering the cut-off points, however, would dramatically increase the number of individuals classified as overweight and obese worldwide.

The sensitivity to develop diabetes, particularly in these populations, is probably one of the main reasons why King et al [43] projected that most of the increase in the prevalence of T2DM is expected to be in developing countries. In 2030, the countries that will have the largest numbers of individuals who have diabetes will be India, China, and the United States.

Even only moderately overweight is closely related to the onset of T2DM. Among British men aged 40 to 59 years who were followed for a mean period of 12 years, weight loss of more than 4% during the first 5 years of follow-up showed a 1.5-times reduced risk for developing T2DM compared with that in men who had stable weight [41]. In a 4-year, double-blind, prospective, randomized study involving 3305 patients, 2.8 kg weight loss decreased the incidence of diabetes from 9.0% to 6.2% [44]. In a recent meta-analysis on bariatric surgery, diabetes was completely resolved in 76.8% of patients and resolved or improved in 86% [45].

Metabolic syndrome and type II diabetes mellitus in children and adolescents

Alarming data from the United States were published [46] in the late 1990s suggesting that the epidemic of pediatric obesity is being followed by an increase in the incidence and prevalence of T2DM. The American Diabetes Association has issued a consensus statement on T2DM in youth, stating that 845% of children newly diagnosed as having diabetes mellitus had a type of diabetes that was not the typical type I diabetes mellitus, based on immune injury to the pancreas in childhood, but rather the type of diabetes traditionally called "adult diabetes" [47]. The phenomenon of a rapidly rising incidence of T2DM in young patients is well known in North America [46]. T2DM now accounts for as many as 8% to 46% of new cases of pediatric diabetes and affects up to 5% of adolescents in some Native American tribes [46,48].

Obesity and cardiovascular disease

Obesity has been associated with many co-occurring cardiovascular disease (CVD) risk factors and CVD mortality. According to Kannel [49], no risk factor has as strong an impact on the cardiovascular risk profile as obesity.

Abdominal adiposity in particular is associated with CVD risk [50–53]. Obesity is a risk factor for increased blood pressure and an unfavorable lipid profile, including decreased high-density lipoprotein cholesterol level and increased low-density lipoprotein cholesterol and triglyceride levels [54]. Weight loss has been shown to improve blood pressure, lipid levels, and diabetes [45,55,56]. Increased blood pressure or unfavorable lipid levels are related to CVD [57,58]. However, obesity is also directly related to CVD independent of blood pressure and lipid levels [26]. That is, when adjustments are made for blood pressure and cholesterol levels, the relationship between obesity and CVD is attenuated, but relative risks remain high and significant [50,59].

The age-adjusted relative risk for incident coronary heart disease (CHD) among men and women is higher than the relative risk for high BMI for mortality. United States women from the Nurses' Health Study [60] who had a BMI above 30 kg/m^2 had a threefold risk for developing nonfatal myocardial infarction compared with women who had a BMI below 21 kg/m^2. Among men in the Health Professionals Study [61], those who had a BMI between 29 and 33 kg/m^2 had a twofold risk, and those who had a BMI higher than 33 kg/m^2 had a threefold risk for developing CHD compared with men who had a BMI below 23 kg/m^2. Among these men and women, high BMI was also related to the onset of stroke [53,62]. The Nurses' Health Study reported that high BMI levels were especially related to the onset of ischemic stroke. Hemorrhagic strokes, which occur less often than ischemic strokes, appear to be less common in those who have a high BMI compared with those whose BMI is low [62].

Data from the Framingham Heart Study, based on 26 years of follow-up of approximately 5200 men and women aged 28 to 62 years, showed that high relative weights were predictive of myocardial infarction, sudden death, congestive heart failure, and atherothrombolic strokes [26]. The British Regional Heart Study of 7700 men aged 40–59 years, followed for a mean period of 14.8 years, showed that high BMI levels were related to incident coronary heart events and, although to a lesser extent, stroke [59].

The association between BMI and the risk for developing atrial fibrillation was examined in a prospective, community-based observational cohort in Framingham, Massachusetts that included 5282 participants [63]. Adjusted for cardiovascular risk factors and interim myocardial infarction or heart failure, a 4% increase in atrial fibrillation risk per one-unit increase in BMI was observed in men and in women. Adjusted hazard ratios for atrial fibrillation associated with obesity were 1.52 and 1.46 for men and women, respectively, compared with individuals who had normal BMI.

Obesity and musculoskeletal disorders

Excess body weight is a well-established risk factor for several types of arthritis, including OA [64–68], rheumatoid arthritis (RA) [69–71], and gout

[72]. Not only is excess weight a primary risk factor for the development of arthritis [68,69,73], but it also increases the risk for disease progression [74,75] and disability among people who have arthritis [74–76]. In addition, people who have disabilities are 2.5 times more likely to be obese than those who do not have such disabilities [77]. Among adults who have lower extremity mobility disabilities, 24.9% were obese versus 15.1% of those who do not have these disabilities. A shift from normal to overweight may carry a higher risk for knee OA requiring arthroplasty than does constant overweight [68].

Knee arthritis is directly related to body weight. Relative to a BMI of 24.0 to 24.9 kg/m^2, the risk for knee OA increased progressively from 0.1 for a BMI less than 20 kg/m^2 to 13.6 for a BMI of 36 kg/m^2 or more. If all overweight and obese people reduced their weight by 5 kg or until their BMI was within the recommended normal range, 24% of surgical cases of knee OA might be avoided [78]. The relationship between being overweight and having OA is explained, at least in part, by the high joint pressure in overweight individuals. There might also be a metabolic explanation, because obesity seems to be related to incident OA in the hands [79].

Serum uric acid concentration showed positive associations with BMI [72]. The size of the visceral fat area was the strongest contributor to an elevated serum concentration of uric acid, a decrease in uric acid clearance, and an increase in the urinary uric acid/creatinine ratio [80].

Two population-based case control studies have shown an association between obesity (BMI > 30) and the development of RA [70,71]. The association appears to be a threshold effect with no relationship between BMI and risk for RA below a BMI of 30.

Obesity and cancer

In a recent study from a prospective cancer prevention cohort, it was estimated that overweight and obesity account for 14% of all cancer deaths in men and 20% of those in women [35]. Significant positive associations were found between obesity and higher death rates for the following cancers: esophagus; colon and rectum; liver; gallbladder; pancreas; kidney; stomach (in men); prostate; breast; uterus; cervix; and ovary. The authors estimated that over 90,000 cancer deaths per year could be avoided if the adult population all maintained a normal weight (BMI < 25). Obesity is clearly a major risk factor for cancer.

Breast cancer

Breast cancer is the most common cancer occurring among women in the United States, accounting for nearly one of every three cancers diagnosed and more than 40,000 deaths in 2003 [81]. Breast cancer risks are often discussed separately for occurrence pre- and postmenopause. In the Nurses'

Health Study, a total of 47,382 United States registered nurses who reported their waist and hip circumferences in 1986 were followed up through May 1994. The waist circumference was nonsignificantly related to risk for premenopausal breast cancer but was significantly associated with post-menopausal breast cancer after adjustment for established breast cancer risk factors [82]. The same group also reported that weight gain after the age of 18 years was unrelated to breast cancer incidence before menopause, but was positively associated with incidence after menopause [83].

The Women's Health Initiative Observational Study followed 85,917 women aged 50 to 79 years. Among hormone replacement therapy (HRT) nonusers, heavier women (baseline BMI > 31.1) had an elevated risk for postmenopausal breast cancer (relative risk = 2.52) compared with slimmer women (baseline BMI < 22.6). Change in BMI since 18 years of age, maximum BMI, and weight were also associated with breast cancer in HRT nonusers [28]. Findings from the European prospective investigation into cancer and nutrition (EPIC) study in Europe confirm that weight, BMI, and hip circumference were positively associated with breast cancer risk. Obese women (BMI > 30) had a 31% excess risk compared with women who had a BMI less than 25 [84].

A population-based, case-control study found that weight change and obesity are risk factors for breast cancer in Hispanic and non-Hispanic white women. However, the risk for Hispanic women is evident independent of menopausal status, whereas the risk for non-Hispanics is apparent in postmenopausal women [85].

The relationship between BMI and postmenopausal breast cancer mortality was examined in the American Cancer Society's Cancer Prevention Study II [86]. Breast cancer mortality rates increased continually and substantially with increasing BMI from 18.5 to 20.49 to more than 40. Approximately 30% to 50% of breast cancer deaths among postmeno-pausal women in the United States population are attributable to overweight.

Recent results from a multicenter trial show that risk for contralateral breast cancer was elevated in obese women who had a history of breast cancer compared with women of normal weight who had breast cancer, independent of tamoxifen use. These results suggest that the effect of obesity may be cumulative and exacerbated to influence tumor development despite treatment after diagnosis of the first primary [87].

Increased risk from weight gain was largely restricted to women who were lean at age 18 years and those who had ER+/PR+ tumors. The elevated odds ratio (OR) was strongest for ER+ and PR+ breast cancer among postmenopausal Hispanic, non-Hispanic white women, and Japa-nese women who had a high BMI [85,88].

The increase in breast cancer risk with increasing BMI among postmenopausal women is largely the result of the associated increase in estrogens, particularly bioavailable estradiol [89].

Most of the relevant prospective studies support an inverse relationship between BMI and the relative risk for developing premenopausal breast cancer [90]. However, some studies have reported a positive relationship between obesity and premenopausal breast cancer when there is family history of breast cancer [91,92].

Prostate cancer

Prostate cancer is the most common noncutaneous malignancy in men, representing 33% of all newly diagnosed cancers, with 230,000 new cases and 30,000 deaths expected in 2004 [93]. Studies examining the relationship between adult BMI and risk for developing prostate cancer have been mixed, with several large studies showing a positive association [94–97] and others showing no association [98,99]. Of the studies that found a significant association between increased BMI and risk for developing prostate cancer, several found that the risk for developing advanced disease was even stronger than the risk for developing prostate cancer in general [95,97]. Visceral obesity may play an important role in the link between obesity and development of prostate cancer. One study among men in China found that men in the highest quartile of waist-to-hip ratio had an almost threefold increased risk for developing prostate cancer [100].

Although the relationship between obesity and prostate cancer risk is unclear, the relationship between obesity and progression and mortality from prostate cancer is well established [27,97,101,102]. Two recent studies used large multi-institutional, multiracial databases to address whether increased BMI was associated with higher biochemical failure rates following radical prostatectomy [103,104]. Both studies concluded that obese men were more likely to have higher-grade disease and that obesity was an independent predictor of prostate cancer recurrence following radical prostatectomy. Both studies found that black men were more likely to be obese, which may partly explain the higher mortality from prostate cancer among black men.

Regarding obesity and prostate cancer mortality, two large prospective studies deserve particular attention. In 1959 and again in 1982, the American Cancer Society enrolled a cohort of patients for longitudinal studies on cancer, known as the Cancer Prevention Study (CPS) I and II, respectively. Men were followed for 13 years in CPS-I and 14 years in CPS-II. Together these studies followed a total of 816,268 men, during which time there were 5212 prostate cancer deaths. CPS-I and CPS-II reported that obese men (BMI $> 30 \text{ kg/m}^2$) were significantly more likely to die from prostate cancer, with a 27% increased risk for prostate cancer death from CPS-I and a 21% increased risk for death from CPS-II [101]. More details regarding CPS-II were recently published that show that severely obese men (BMI $> 35 \text{ kg/m}^2$) had a 34% higher risk of dying from prostate cancer relative to normal-weight men [27].

Uterine cancer

The relationship of obesity to an increased risk for uterine cancer is well established [105–110]. In a case-control study in western New York State [111], interviews were conducted with 232 incident endometrial cancer patients diagnosed between 1986 and 1991, and 631 community controls were examined to determine the effects of obesity at times before the diagnosis of uterine cancer. BMI at 16 years of age and 20, 10, and 2 years before interview, and changes in BMI between these periods were examined. Although being heavy at 16 years of age was associated with slightly increased risk (adjusted OR, 1.28; 95% confidence interval [CI], 0.84–1.96), large gains over the entire period from 16 years of age to 2 years before diagnosis (OR, 3.45; CI, 2.13–5.57) and high BMI close to the time of diagnosis (OR, 3.21; CI, 2.01–5.15) were associated with greater risk. Differences in mean BMI between cases and controls increased over time.

In a case-cohort study, 62,573 women from The Netherlands Cohort Study on Diet and Cancer were followed up from 1986 to 1995, and 226 endometrial cancer case patients were identified [105]. Compared with women who had a BMI between 20 and 22.9, women who had a BMI of 30 or greater had a higher risk for endometrial cancer (relative risk = 4.50). Moreover, BMI at 20 years of age and BMI gain since 20 years of age were positively associated with endometrial cancer risk.

In a population-based, case-control study conducted in urban Shanghai, obesity in adulthood was associated with elevated risks, with ORs for the highest versus lowest quartile of BMI being 1.5, 1.7, 1.9, and 1.7 at ages 30, 40, 50, and 60, respectively. Weight gain of more than 7.5 kg at different 10-year intervals in adulthood was associated with increased risk for endometrial cancer. Only weight loss from ages 20 to 30 years was inversely associated with endometrial cancer risk [106].

Ovarian cancer

In the United States, ovarian cancer is the fourth most frequent cause of cancer death among women, following lung, breast, and colorectal cancers. Each year, approximately 26,000 women are diagnosed with ovarian cancer and 14,000 die. The relationship between BMI and ovarian cancer mortality was examined among postmenopausal women in a large prospective mortality study of 300,537 women who were cancer-free at enrollment in 1982 and had no history of hysterectomy or ovarian surgery. During 16 years of follow-up, 1511 deaths occurred from ovarian cancer. Ovarian cancer mortality rates were higher among overweight (BMI ≥ 25) and obese women (BMI ≥ 30) compared with women who had a BMI less than 25 [112]. A population-based study of 563 cases of ovarian cancer and 523 controls found that weight and BMI were associated positively with risk among premenopausal women, but did not affect risk postmenopausally.

High BMI, weight, and height were most strongly related to risk for serous borderline cancer, particularly among premenopausal women [113].

A case-control study was conducted to assess environmental and other risk factors for ovarian cancer from 1994 to 1996 in northern Kyushu, Japan [114]. Among 89 cases of women who had epithelial ovarian cancer and 323 controls who did not have any cancer or ovarian disorder, the ORs of ovarian cancer across increasing quartiles of the heaviest body weight were 1, 1.15, 1.71, and 2.29 ($P = .008$, test for trend). This study provides additional support for an association between obesity and the risk for ovarian cancer. Other studies, however, have found no association between obesity and ovarian cancer [115]. Additional research on the exact mechanisms underlying this association is needed.

Renal cell cancer

Obesity has also been associated with an increased risk for renal cell cancer. In a multicenter, population-based, case-control study concerning incident cases of histologic, verified renal cell cancer ($N = 1732$) and age- and sex-matched controls ($N = 2309$), BMI was found to be a risk factor among women and, to a lesser extent, among men. A threefold increased risk (relative risk, 3.6; 95% CI, 2.3–5.7) was observed for women who had a relative weight in the top 5% compared with those whose weight was in the lowest quartile. Rate of weight change (estimated as weight change per annum in kilograms) appeared to be an independent risk factor among women but not among men [116].

In a population-based, case-control study [117] that included 449 directly interviewed cases and 707 controls, risk for renal cell carcinoma increased with increasing BMI among women. A nearly fourfold risk was found among the 10% of women who had the highest BMI (OR, 3.8; CI, 1.7–8.4). Among men, no clear trend was observed with usual weight or BMI, although the highest risk (30%–50%) generally was seen among those who were in the upper deciles of weight or BMI.

The associations of obesity with an increased risk for renal cell cancer among women, although weaker in men, have been shown by the above studies and several other studies [118]. However, a quantitative summary analysis, including all studies examining body weight in relation to kidney cancer available in MEDLINE from 1966 to 1998, found the relative risk estimate was 1.07 (95% CI, 1.05–1.09) per unit of increase in BMI (corresponding to 3-kg body weight increase for a subject of average height) among men and women [119]. There was no evidence of effect modification by sex [119]. A recent population control study in Canada found an increased risk for renal cell carcinoma associated with overweight and obesity among male and female adults [120].

Obesity and hypertension have also been implicated as risk factors for the development of renal cell cancer in men. Compared with men in the lowest three eighths of the cohort for BMI, men in the middle three eighths had a 30% to 60% greater risk for renal-cell cancer, and men in the highest two eighths had nearly double the risk. After the first 5 years of follow-up had been excluded to reduce possible effects of preclinical disease, the risk for renal-cell cancer was still consistently higher in men who had a higher BMI or higher blood pressure. At the 6-year follow-up, the risk rose further with increasing blood pressures and decreased with decreasing blood pressures, after adjustment for baseline measurements [121].

Colon cancer

Obesity has been reported to increase the risk for colon cancer, especially in men. The American Cancer Society's Cancer Prevention Study II [122], a nationwide mortality study of United States adults, documented 1616 deaths from colon cancer in women and 1792 in men over 12 years of follow-up among 496,239 women and 379,167 men who were cancer-free at enrollment in 1982. In men, death rates from colon cancer increased across the entire range of BMI. The rate ratio was highest for men who had a BMI of 32.5 or more (rate ratio, 1.90; 95% CI, 1.46–2.47) compared with men who had a BMI between 22 and 23.49. In women, a weaker association was seen in the three BMI categories of 27.5 to 29.9 (rate ratio, 1.26; 95% CI, 1.03–1.53), 30 to 32.4 (rate ratio, 1.37; 95% CI, 1.09–1.72), and 32.5 or more (rate ratio, 1.23; 95% CI, 0.96–1.59).

Further evidence that obesity increases the risk for colon cancer and adenomas, which are precursors of cancer, and that an abdominal distribution of obesity is an independent risk factor for these events was obtained in a study of 47,723 male health professionals [123]. BMI was directly associated with risk for colon cancer independent of physical activity level. Waist circumference and waist/hip ratio were strong risk factors for colon cancer (waist/hip ratio ≥0.99 compared with waist/hip ratio <0.90: multivariate relative risk, 3.41 [CI, 1.52–7.66], $P =.01$; waist circumference ≥43 in compared with waist circumference <35 in: relative risk, 2.56 [CI, 1.33–4.96], $P < .001$). These associations persisted even after adjustment for BMI.

Pancreatic cancer

In a population-based, case-control study in seven of the ten Canadian provinces, 312 patients who had histologically confirmed pancreatic cancer were compared with 2919 controls. Men in the highest quartile of BMI (≥28.3) were at increased risk for pancreatic cancer (adjusted OR, 1.90; 95% CI, 1.08–3.35) [124]. In two prospective United States cohort studies, individuals who had a BMI of at least 30 kg/m^2 had an elevated risk for pancreatic cancer compared with those who had a BMI of less than 23 (multivariable relative risk, 1.72; 95% CI, 1.19–2.48) [125].

In a study designed to examine the possible role of body size and reproductive factors in pancreatic cancer, data were analyzed from a population-based, case-control study conducted in Shanghai, China [126]. After adjustment for age, income, smoking, and other confounders, a positive dose-response relation between BMI and risk for pancreatic cancer was observed in both sexes.

A recent meta-analysis from published data from 1966 to 2003 included six case-control and eight cohort studies involving 6391 cases of pancreatic cancer [127]. The estimated per unit increase in BMI would translate into a relative risk of 1.19 (95% CI, 1.10–1.29) for obese people (BMI > 30) compared with people who have a normal body weight (BMI = 22). These results provide evidence that the risk for pancreatic cancer may be weakly associated with obesity. However, the small magnitude of the summary risk means the possibility of confounding cannot be excluded.

Pulmonary complications of obesity

Obesity can have profound adverse effects on the respiratory system. It can cause alterations in respiratory mechanics, respiratory muscle strength and endurance, pulmonary gas exchange, control of breathing, pulmonary function tests, and exercise capacity. Common complaints include dyspnea on exertion and exercise intolerance. Obese persons are at increased risk for developing respiratory complications such as atelectasis, severe hypoxemia, pulmonary embolism, aspiration pneumonia, and acute ventilatory failure, particularly in the perioperative and postoperative periods [128].

In a cross-sectional representative survey of 5887 men and 7018 women aged 20 to 59 years from the Netherlands, the ORs for shortness of breath when walking upstairs in individuals who had a BMI of 30 or higher were 3.5 in men and 3.3 in women after adjustments for age and lifestyle factors [129].

A subgroup of obese persons develops chronic daytime hypoventilation, defined as a sustained increase in arterial carbon dioxide tension exceeding 45 mm Hg. Those who do are typically extremely obese. The term *obesity hypoventilation syndrome* (OHS) is used to describe this combination of severe obesity and diurnal hypoventilation. Obese persons who do not have OHS are said to have simple or uncomplicated obesity.

Sharp et al [130] reported in the 1960s that in simple or uncomplicated obesity, chest wall and total respiratory system compliance were 92% and 80%, respectively, of predicted normal values. These values were substantially lower in patients who had OHS whose chest wall and total respiratory system compliance were 37% and 44% of normal, respectively. This decrement in total respiratory system compliance is at least partially caused by a fall in lung compliance, which is decreased by approximately 25% in simple obesity and 40% in OHS [130,131].

Obesity is also the most common predisposing factor to obstructive sleep apnea (OSA) syndrome. If BMI is defined as more than 28 kg/m^2, obesity is present in 60% to 90% of OSA patients evaluated in sleep clinics [132–135]. In one investigation, an increase in BMI of 1 SD was associated with a fourfold increase in risk for OSA [136]. In another study, obesity was a better predictor of severity of sleep apnea than gender and age [132]. However, there is evidence that the distribution of fat, in particular upper body obesity, rather than total body fat is most important to the development of OSA syndrome [137,138].

Numerous studies have indicated that OSA generally improves with weight loss [139–141]. A recent meta-analysis on bariatric surgery, including a total of 136 fully extracted studies, reported that the percentage of patients in the total study population whose OSA resolved was 85.7% (95% CI, 79.2%–92.2%). The percentage of patients in the total population whose OSA resolved or improved was 83.6% (95% CI, 71.8%–95.4%) [45].

Cost for treating obesity-related medical conditions

The increasing prevalence of obesity in the United States is alarming, especially as it translates into increased medical care and disability costs. Approximately $51.6 billion of these costs were direct medical costs associated with diseases attributable to obesity annually. This amount represented 5.7% of the total national health care expenditures of the United States. The indirect costs attributable to obesity have been estimated at $47.6 billion. Indirect costs represent the value of lost work caused by morbidity and mortality and may have a greater impact than direct costs at the personal and societal levels [142].

In 1999, Colditz [143] reported that the direct and indirect costs of obesity were estimated to be 7% of the total health care costs in the United States and between 1% to 5% in Europe [144]. These estimates were based on prevalence rates and relative risks. Because of its closer relationship to morbidity and disability than mortality, obesity will enormously increase the number of unhealthy life years.

The total direct cost of obesity in Canada in 1997 was estimated to be over $1.8 billion. This amount corresponded to 2.4% of the total health care expenditures for all diseases in Canada in 1997. When the contributions of the comorbidities to the total cost were considered, the three largest contributors were hypertension ($656.6 million), T2DM ($423.2 million), and coronary artery disease ($346.0 million) [145].

Oster and colleagues [146] calculated that weight loss of about 10% of initial body weight would reduce the number of life years spent suffering from hypertension by 1.2 to 2.9 years and from T2DM by 0.5 to 1.7 years. Life expectancy would be increased by 27 months. Again, these estimates are based on calculations using relative risks for the specific outcomes. Empiric data on how many more years obese persons spend suffering from morbidity and disability than do normal-weight persons have yet to be published.

Summary

Obesity and overweight account for a substantial percentage of overall health care costs and contribute significantly to morbidity and mortality in the United States and around the world. For the first time in human history, the numbers of overweight and underweight individuals are about the same, at 2.1 billion each. More disturbing than simply those figures is the explosion of obesity and overweight with related health problems around the world. In many countries, overweight coexists with poverty-related malnutrition in what is called the "nutrition transition." This phenomenon occurs often as Western foods and lifestyles are introduced in many foreign lands. A worldwide strategy for combating obesity and its causes, including modification of the food supply and reducing the obesogenic environment by increasing opportunities in daily life for physical activity and structured exercise, is a high priority for individuals and governments worldwide. Prevention is clearly more cost-effective than treatment of obesity and should be instituted beginning with the world's children.

References

[1] Bray GA, Greenway FL. Current and potential drugs for treatment of obesity. Endocr Rev 1999;20(6):805–75.

[2] Flegal KM, Carroll MD, Ogden CL, et al. Prevalence and trends in obesity among US adults, 1999–2000. JAMA 2002;288(14):1723–7.

[3] World Health Organization. Controlling the global obesity epidemic, 1985–1998. Available at: http//www.who.int/nut/obs.html. Accessed June 20, 2003.

[4] Mokdad AH, Serdula MK, Dietz WH, et al. The spread of the obesity epidemic in the United States, 1991–1998. JAMA 1999;282(16):1519–22.

[5] Mokdad AH, Serdula MK, Dietz WH, et al. The continuing epidemic of obesity in the United States. JAMA 2000;284(13):1650–1.

[6] Mokdad AH, Bowman BA, Ford ES, et al. The continuing epidemics of obesity and diabetes in the United States. JAMA 2001;286(10):1195–200.

[7] Mokdad AH, Ford ES, Bowman BA, et al. Prevalence of obesity, diabetes, and obesity-related health risk factors 2001. JAMA 2003;289(1):76–9.

[8] Kuczmarski RJ, Flegal KM, Campbell SM, et al. Increasing prevalence of overweight among US adults. The National Health and Nutrition Examination Surveys, 1960 to 1991. JAMA 1994;272(3):205–11.

[9] Kuczmarski RJ, Carroll MD, Flegal KM, et al. Varying body mass index cutoff points to describe overweight prevalence among US adults: NHANES III (1988 to 1994). Obes Res 1997;5(6):542–8.

[10] Centers for Disease Control and Prevention. Obesity epidemic increases dramatically in the United States. Available at: http//www.cdc.gov/nccdphp/dnpa/obeistyepidemichim. Accessed June 11, 2002.

[11] U.S.Department of Health and Human Services. Healthy people 2010. 2nd edition [report]. Washington (DC): US Government Printing Office; 2000.

[12] U.S. Department of Health and Human Services. The Surgeon General's call to action to prevent and decrease overweight and obesity [pamphlet]. Rockville (MD): U.S. Department of Health and Human Services; 2001.

[13] Ryan AS, Roche AF, Kuczmarski RJ. Weight, stature, and body mass index data for Mexican Americans from the third national health and nutrition examination survey (NHANES III, 1988–1994). Am J Human Biol 1999;11(5):673–86.

[14] Katzmarzyk PT. The Canadian obesity epidemic: an historical perspective. Obes Res 2002; 10(7):666–74.

[15] Canning PM, Courage ML, Frizzell LM. Prevalence of overweight and obesity in a provincial population of Canadian preschool children. CMAJ 2004;171(3):240–2.

[16] Friedrich MJ. Epidemic of obesity expands its spread to developing countries. JAMA 2002; 287(11):1382–6.

[17] Seidell JC, Flegal KM. Assessing obesity: classification and epidemiology. Br Med Bull 1997;53(2):238–52.

[18] Molarius A, Seidell JC, Sans S, et al. Educational level, relative body weight, and changes in their association over 10 years: an international perspective from the WHO MONICA Project. Am J Public Health 2000;90(8):1260–8.

[19] Seidell JC. Obesity, insulin resistance and diabetes–a worldwide epidemic. Br J Nutr 2000; 83(Suppl 1):S5–8.

[20] World Health Organization. Life in the 21st Century—a vision for all. The World Health Report. Geneva, Switzerland: World Health Organization; 1998.

[21] Bell AC, Ge K, Popkin BM. Weight gain and its predictors in Chinese adults. Int J Obes Relat Metab Disord 2001;25(7):1079–86.

[22] Lissau I, Overpeck MD, Ruan WJ, et al. Body mass index and overweight in adolescents in 13 European countries, Israel, and the United States. Arch Pediatr Adolesc Med 2004; 158(1):27–33.

[23] Cheng TO. Childhood obesity in China. Health Place 2004;10(4):395–6.

[24] Luo J, Hu FB. Time trends of obesity in pre-school children in China from 1989 to 1997. Int J Obes Relat Metab Disord 2002;26(4):553–8.

[25] Iwata F, Hara M, Okada T, et al. Body fat ratios in urban Chinese children. Pediatr Int 2003;45(2):190–2.

[26] Hubert HB, Feinleib M, McNamara PM, et al. Obesity as an independent risk factor for cardiovascular disease: a 26-year follow-up of participants in the Framingham Heart Study. Circulation 1983;67(5):968–77.

[27] Calle EE, Rodriguez C, Walker-Thurmond K, et al. Overweight, obesity, and mortality from cancer in a prospectively studied cohort of US adults. N Engl J Med 2003;348(17): 1625–38.

[28] Morimoto LM, White E, Chen Z, et al. Obesity, body size, and risk of postmenopausal breast cancer: the Women's Health Initiative (United States). Cancer Causes Control 2002; 13(8):741–51.

[29] Lindstrom J, Eriksson JG, Valle TT, et al. Prevention of diabetes mellitus in subjects with impaired glucose tolerance in the Finnish Diabetes Prevention Study: results from a randomized clinical trial. J Am Soc Nephrol 2003;14(7 Suppl 2):S108–13.

[30] Sjostrom LV. Mortality of severely obese subjects. Am J Clin Nutr 1992;55(Suppl 2): S516–23.

[31] Manson JE, Stampfer MJ, Hennekens CH, et al. Body weight and longevity. A reassessment. JAMA 1987;257(3):353–8.

[32] Manson JE, Willett WC, Stampfer MJ, et al. Body weight and mortality among women. N Engl J Med 1995;333(11):677–85.

[33] Baik I, Ascherio A, Rimm EB, et al. Adiposity and mortality in men. Am J Epidemiol 2000; 152(3):264–71.

[34] Ajani UA, Lotufo PA, Gaziano JM, et al. Body mass index and mortality among US male physicians. Ann Epidemiol 2004;14(10):731–9.

[35] Calle EE, Thun MJ, Petrelli JM, et al. Body-mass index and mortality in a prospective cohort of US adults. N Engl J Med 1999;341(15):1097–105.

[36] Willett WC, Dietz WH, Colditz GA. Guidelines for healthy weight. N Engl J Med 1999; 341(6):427–34.

[37] Moore B. Shape-up America [report]. 2004.

[38] Harris MI. Epidemiologic studies on the pathogenesis of non-insulin-dependent diabetes mellitus (NIDDM). Clin Invest Med 1995;18(4):231–9.

[39] Chan JM, Rimm EB, Colditz GA, et al. Obesity, fat distribution, and weight gain as risk factors for clinical diabetes in men. Diabetes Care 1994;17(9):961–9.

[40] Colditz GA, Willett WC, Stampfer MJ, et al. Weight as a risk factor for clinical diabetes in women. Am J Epidemiol 1990;132(3):501–13.

[41] Wannamethee SG, Shaper AG. Weight change and duration of overweight and obesity in the incidence of type 2 diabetes. Diabetes Care 1999;22(8):1266–72.

[42] Kosaka K, Kuzuya T, Yoshinaga H, et al. A prospective study of health check examinees for the development of non-insulin-dependent diabetes mellitus: relationship of the incidence of diabetes with the initial insulinogenic index and degree of obesity. Diabet Med 1996;13(9 Suppl 6):S120–6.

[43] King H, Aubert RE, Herman WH. Global burden of diabetes, 1995–2025: prevalence, numerical estimates, and projections. Diabetes Care 1998;21(9):1414–31.

[44] Torgerson JS, Hauptman J, Boldrin MN, et al. XENical in the prevention of diabetes in obese subjects (XENDOS) study: a randomized study of orlistat as an adjunct to lifestyle changes for the prevention of type 2 diabetes in obese patients. Diabetes Care 2004;27(1): 155–61.

[45] Buchwald H, Avidor Y, Braunwald E, et al. Bariatric surgery: a systematic review and meta-analysis. JAMA 2004;292(14):1724–37.

[46] Pinhas-Hamiel O, Dolan LM, Daniels SR, et al. Increased incidence of non-insulin-dependent diabetes mellitus among adolescents. J Pediatr 1996;128(5 Pt 1):608–15.

[47] American Diabetes Association. Type 2 diabetes in children and adolescents. Pediatrics 2000;105(3 Pt 1):671–80.

[48] Fagot-Campagna A, Pettitt DJ, Engelgau MM, et al. Type 2 diabetes among North American children and adolescents: an epidemiologic review and a public health perspective. J Pediatr 2000;136(5):664–72.

[49] Kannel WB. Effect of weight on cardiovascular disease. Nutrition 1997;13(2):157–8.

[50] Donahue RP, Abbott RD, Bloom E, et al. Central obesity and coronary heart disease in men. Lancet 1987;1(8537):821–4.

[51] Gray RS, Fabsitz RR, Cowan LD, et al. Relation of generalized and central obesity to cardiovascular risk factors and prevalent coronary heart disease in a sample of American Indians: the Strong Heart Study. Int J Obes Relat Metab Disord 2000;24(7): 849–60.

[52] Rexrode KM, Buring JE, Manson JE. Abdominal and total adiposity and risk of coronary heart disease in men. Int J Obes Relat Metab Disord 2001;25(7):1047–56.

[53] Walker SP, Rimm EB, Ascherio A, et al. Body size and fat distribution as predictors of stroke among US men. Am J Epidemiol 1996;144(12):1143–50.

[54] Despres JP, Tremblay A, Perusse L, et al. Abdominal adipose tissue and serum HDL-cholesterol: association independent from obesity and serum triglyceride concentration. Int J Obes 1988;12(1):1–13.

[55] Ashley FW Jr, Kannel WB. Relation of weight change to changes in atherogenic traits: the Framingham Study. J Chronic Dis 1974;27(3):103–14.

[56] Dattilo AM, Kris-Etherton PM. Effects of weight reduction on blood lipids and lipoproteins: a meta-analysis. Am J Clin Nutr 1992;56(2):320–8.

[57] van den Hoogen PC, Feskens EJ, Nagelkerke NJ, et al. The relation between blood pressure and mortality due to coronary heart disease among men in different parts of the world. Seven Countries Study Research Group. N Engl J Med 2000;342(1):1–8.

[58] Verschuren WM, Jacobs DR, Bloemberg BP, et al. Serum total cholesterol and long-term coronary heart disease mortality in different cultures. Twenty-five-year follow-up of the seven countries study. JAMA 1995;274(2):131–6.

[59] Shaper AG, Wannamethee SG, Walker M. Body weight: implications for the prevention of coronary heart disease, stroke, and diabetes mellitus in a cohort study of middle aged men. BMJ 1997;314(7090):1311–7.

[60] Manson JE, Colditz GA, Stampfer MJ, et al. A prospective study of obesity and risk of coronary heart disease in women. N Engl J Med 1990;322(13):882–9.

[61] Rimm EB, Stampfer MJ, Giovannucci E, et al. Body size and fat distribution as predictors of coronary heart disease among middle-aged and older US men. Am J Epidemiol 1995; 141(12):1117–27.

[62] Rexrode KM, Hennekens CH, Willett WC, et al. A prospective study of body mass index, weight change, and risk of stroke in women. JAMA 1997;277(19):1539–45.

[63] Wang TJ, Parise H, Levy D, et al. Obesity and the risk of new-onset atrial fibrillation. JAMA 2004;292(20):2471–7.

[64] Carman WJ, Sowers M, Hawthorne VM, et al. Obesity as a risk factor for osteoarthritis of the hand and wrist: a prospective study. Am J Epidemiol 1994;139(2):119–29.

[65] Gelber AC, Hochberg MC, Mead LA, et al. Body mass index in young men and the risk of subsequent knee and hip osteoarthritis. Am J Med 1999;107(6):542–8.

[66] Hart DJ, Spector TD. The relationship of obesity, fat distribution and osteoarthritis in women in the general population: the Chingford Study. J Rheumatol 1993;20(2):331–5.

[67] Hochberg MC, Lethbridge-Cejku M, Scott WW Jr, et al. The association of body weight, body fatness and body fat distribution with osteoarthritis of the knee: data from the Baltimore Longitudinal Study of Aging. J Rheumatol 1995;22(3):488–93.

[68] Manninen P, Riihimaki H, Heliovaara M, et al. Weight changes and the risk of knee osteoarthritis requiring arthroplasty. Ann Rheum Dis 2004;63(11):1434–7.

[69] Symmons DP. Epidemiology of rheumatoid arthritis: determinants of onset, persistence and outcome. Best Pract Res Clin Rheumatol 2002;16(5):707–22.

[70] Symmons DP, Bankhead CR, Harrison BJ, et al. Blood transfusion, smoking, and obesity as risk factors for the development of rheumatoid arthritis: results from a primary care-based incident case-control study in Norfolk, England. Arthritis Rheum 1997;40(11): 1955–61.

[71] Voigt LF, Koepsell TD, Nelson JL, et al. Smoking, obesity, alcohol consumption, and the risk of rheumatoid arthritis. Epidemiology 1994;5(5):525–32.

[72] Roubenoff R, Klag MJ, Mead LA, et al. Incidence and risk factors for gout in white men. JAMA 1991;266(21):3004–7.

[73] Felson DT, Zhang Y, Hannan MT, et al. Risk factors for incident radiographic knee osteoarthritis in the elderly: the Framingham Study. Arthritis Rheum 1997;40(4):728–33.

[74] Verbrugge LM, Gates DM, Ike RW. Risk factors for disability among US adults with arthritis. J Clin Epidemiol 1991;44(2):167–82.

[75] Felson DT, Lawrence RC, Dieppe PA, et al. Osteoarthritis: new insights. Part 1: the disease and its risk factors. Ann Intern Med 2000;133(8):635–46.

[76] Visser M, Langlois J, Guralnik JM, et al. High body fatness, but not low fat-free mass, predicts disability in older men and women: the Cardiovascular Health Study. Am J Clin Nutr 1998;68(3):584–90.

[77] Weil E, Wachterman M, McCarthy EP, et al. Obesity among adults with disabling conditions. JAMA 2002;288(10):1265–8.

[78] Coggon D, Reading I, Croft P, et al. Knee osteoarthritis and obesity. Int J Obes Relat Metab Disord 2001;25(5):622–7.

[79] Oliveria SA, Felson DT, Cirillo PA, et al. Body weight, body mass index, and incident symptomatic osteoarthritis of the hand, hip, and knee. Epidemiology 1999;10(2):161–6.

[80] Takahashi S, Yamamoto T, Tsutsumi Z, et al. Close correlation between visceral fat accumulation and uric acid metabolism in healthy men. Metabolism 1997;46(10):1162–5.

[81] American Cancer Society. Breast cancer facts and figures 2003–2004. Atlanta, GA: American Cancer Society [report]. 2003.

[82] Huang Z, Willett WC, Colditz GA, et al. Waist circumference, waist:hip ratio, and risk of breast cancer in the Nurses' Health Study. Am J Epidemiol 1999;150(12):1316–24.

[83] Huang Z, Hankinson SE, Colditz GA, et al. Dual effects of weight and weight gain on breast cancer risk. JAMA 1997;278(17):1407–11.

[84] Lahmann PH, Hoffmann K, Allen N, et al. Body size and breast cancer risk: findings from the European Prospective Investigation into Cancer And Nutrition (EPIC). Int J Cancer 2004;111(5):762–71.

[85] Wenten M, Gilliland FD, Baumgartner K, et al. Associations of weight, weight change, and body mass with breast cancer risk in Hispanic and non-Hispanic white women. Ann Epidemiol 2002;12(6):435–44.

[86] Petrelli JM, Calle EE, Rodriguez C, et al. Body mass index, height, and postmenopausal breast cancer mortality in a prospective cohort of US women. Cancer Causes Control 2002; 13(4):325–32.

[87] Dignam JJ, Wieand K, Johnson KA, et al. Obesity, tamoxifen use, and outcomes in women with estrogen receptor-positive early-stage breast cancer. J Natl Cancer Inst 2003;95(19): 1467–76.

[88] Yoo K, Tajima K, Park S, et al. Postmenopausal obesity as a breast cancer risk factor according to estrogen and progesterone receptor status (Japan). Cancer Lett 2001;167(1): 57–63.

[89] Key TJ, Appleby PN, Reeves GK, et al. Body mass index, serum sex hormones, and breast cancer risk in postmenopausal women. J Natl Cancer Inst 2003;95(16):1218–26.

[90] Cleary MP, Maihle NJ. The role of body mass index in the relative risk of developing premenopausal versus postmenopausal breast cancer. Proc Soc Exp Biol Med 1997;216(1): 28–43.

[91] Cerhan JR, Grabrick DM, Vierkant RA, et al. Interaction of adolescent anthropometric characteristics and family history on breast cancer risk in a Historical Cohort Study of 426 families (USA). Cancer Causes Control 2004;15(1):1–9.

[92] Weiderpass E, Braaten T, Magnusson C, et al. A prospective study of body size in different periods of life and risk of premenopausal breast cancer. Cancer Epidemiol Biomarkers Prev 2004;13(7):1121–7.

[93] Jemal A, Clegg LX, Ward E, et al. Annual report to the nation on the status of cancer, 1975–2001, with a special feature regarding survival. Cancer 2004;101(1):3–27.

[94] Engeland A, Tretli S, Bjorge T. Height, body mass index, and prostate cancer: a follow-up of 950000 Norwegian men. Br J Cancer 2003;89(7):1237–42.

[95] Putnam SD, Cerhan JR, Parker AS, et al. Lifestyle and anthropometric risk factors for prostate cancer in a cohort of Iowa men. Ann Epidemiol 2000;10(6):361–9.

[96] Veierod MB, Laake P, Thelle DS. Dietary fat intake and risk of prostate cancer: a prospective study of 25,708 Norwegian men. Int J Cancer 1997;73(5):634–8.

[97] Andersson SO, Wolk A, Bergstrom R, et al. Body size and prostate cancer: a 20-year follow-up study among 135006 Swedish construction workers. J Natl Cancer Inst 1997;89(5): 385–9.

[98] Giovannucci E, Rimm EB, Liu Y, et al. Body mass index and risk of prostate cancer in US health professionals. J Natl Cancer Inst 2003;95(16):1240–4.

[99] Schuurman AG, Goldbohm RA, Dorant E, et al. Anthropometry in relation to prostate cancer risk in the Netherlands Cohort Study. Am J Epidemiol 2000;151(6): 541–9.

[100] Hsing AW, Deng J, Sesterhenn IA, et al. Body size and prostate cancer: a population-based case-control study in China. Cancer Epidemiol Biomarkers Prev 2000;9(12):1335–41.

[101] Rodriguez C, Patel AV, Calle EE, et al. Body mass index, height, and prostate cancer mortality in two large cohorts of adult men in the United States. Cancer Epidemiol Biomarkers Prev 2001;10(4):345–53.

[102] Snowdon DA, Phillips RL, Choi W. Diet, obesity, and risk of fatal prostate cancer. Am J Epidemiol 1984;120(2):244–50.

[103] Amling CL, Riffenburgh RH, Sun L, et al. Pathologic variables and recurrence rates as related to obesity and race in men with prostate cancer undergoing radical prostatectomy. J Clin Oncol 2004;22(3):439–45.

[104] Freedland SJ, Isaacs WB. Explaining racial differences in prostate cancer in the United States: sociology or biology? Prostate 2005;62(3):243–52.

[105] Schouten LJ, Goldbohm RA, van den Brandt PA. Anthropometry, physical activity, and endometrial cancer risk: results from the Netherlands Cohort Study. J Natl Cancer Inst 2004;96(21):1635–8.

[106] Xu W, Dai Q, Ruan Z, et al. Obesity at different ages and endometrial cancer risk factors in urban Shanghai, China. Zhonghua Liu Xing Bing Xue Za Zhi 2002;23(5):347–51.

[107] Shoff SM, Newcomb PA. Diabetes, body size, and risk of endometrial cancer. Am J Epidemiol 1998;148(3):234–40.

[108] Goodman MT, Hankin JH, Wilkens LR, et al. Diet, body size, physical activity, and the risk of endometrial cancer. Cancer Res 1997;57(22):5077–85.

[109] Maggino T, Pirrone F, Velluti F, et al. The role of the endocrine factors and obesity in hormone-dependent gynecological neoplasias. Eur J Gynaecol Oncol 1993;14(2):119–26.

[110] Levi F, La VC, Negri E, et al. Body mass at different ages and subsequent endometrial cancer risk. Int J Cancer 1992;50(4):567–71.

[111] Olson SH, Trevisan M, Marshall JR, et al. Body mass index, weight gain, and risk of endometrial cancer. Nutr Cancer 1995;23(2):141–9.

[112] Rodriguez C, Calle EE, Fakhrabadi-Shokoohi D, et al. Body mass index, height, and the risk of ovarian cancer mortality in a prospective cohort of postmenopausal women. Cancer Epidemiol Biomarkers Prev 2002;11(9):822–8.

[113] Kuper H, Cramer DW, Titus-Ernstoff L. Risk of ovarian cancer in the United States in relation to anthropometric measures: does the association depend on menopausal status? Cancer Causes Control 2002;13(5):455–63.

[114] Mori M, Nishida T, Sugiyama T, et al. Anthropometric and other risk factors for ovarian cancer in a case-control study. Jpn J Cancer Res 1998;89(3):246–53.

[115] Fairfield KM, Willett WC, Rosner BA, et al. Obesity, weight gain, and ovarian cancer. Obstet Gynecol 2002;100(2):288–96.

[116] Mellemgaard A, Lindblad P, Schlehofer B, et al. International renal-cell cancer study. III. Role of weight, height, physical activity, and use of amphetamines. Int J Cancer 1995;60(3): 350–4.

[117] Chow WH, McLaughlin JK, Mandel JS, et al. Obesity and risk of renal cell cancer. Cancer Epidemiol Biomarkers Prev 1996;5(1):17–21.

[118] Lindblad P, Wolk A, Bergstrom R, et al. The role of obesity and weight fluctuations in the etiology of renal cell cancer: a population-based case-control study. Cancer Epidemiol Biomarkers Prev 1994;3(8):631–9.

[119] Bergstrom A, Hsieh CC, Lindblad P, et al. Obesity and renal cell cancer–a quantitative review. Br J Cancer 2001;85(7):984–90.

[120] Hu J, Mao Y, White K. Overweight and obesity in adults and risk of renal cell carcinoma in Canada. Soz Praventivmed 2003;48(3):178–85.

[121] Chow WH, Gridley G, Fraumeni JF Jr, et al. Obesity, hypertension, and the risk of kidney cancer in men. N Engl J Med 2000;343(18):1305–11.

[122] Murphy TK, Calle EE, Rodriguez C, et al. Body mass index and colon cancer mortality in a large prospective study. Am J Epidemiol 2000;152(9):847–54.

[123] Giovannucci E, Ascherio A, Rimm EB, et al. Physical activity, obesity, and risk for colon cancer and adenoma in men. Ann Intern Med 1995;122(5):327–34.

[124] Hanley AJ, Johnson KC, Villeneuve PJ, et al. Physical activity, anthropometric factors and risk of pancreatic cancer: results from the Canadian enhanced cancer surveillance system. Int J Cancer 2001;94(1):140–7.

[125] Michaud DS, Giovannucci E, Willett WC, et al. Physical activity, obesity, height, and the risk of pancreatic cancer. JAMA 2001;286(8):921–9.

[126] Ji BT, Hatch MC, Chow WH, et al. Anthropometric and reproductive factors and the risk of pancreatic cancer: a case-control study in Shanghai, China. Int J Cancer 1996;66(4): 432–7.

[127] Berrington de Gonzalez A, Sweetland S, Spencer E. A meta-analysis of obesity and the risk of pancreatic cancer. Br J Cancer 2003;89(3):519–23.

[128] Koenig SM. Pulmonary complications of obesity. Am J Med Sci 2001;321(4):249–79.

[129] Lean ME, Han TS, Seidell JC. Impairment of health and quality of life using new US federal guidelines for the identification of obesity. Arch Intern Med 1999;159(8):837–43.

[130] Sharp JT, Henry JP, Sweany SK, et al. The total work of breathing in normal and obese men. J Clin Invest 1964;43:728–39.

[131] Pelosi P, Croci M, Ravagnan I, et al. Total respiratory system, lung, and chest wall mechanics in sedated-paralyzed postoperative morbidly obese patients. Chest 1996;109(1): 144–51.

[132] Dealberto MJ, Ferber C, Garma L, et al. Factors related to sleep apnea syndrome in sleep clinic patients. Chest 1994;105(6):1753–8.

[133] van Boxem TJ, de Groot GH. Prevalence and severity of sleep disordered breathing in a group of morbidly obese patients. Neth J Med 1999;54(5):202–6.

[134] Levinson PD, McGarvey ST, Carlisle CC, et al. Adiposity and cardiovascular risk factors in men with obstructive sleep apnea. Chest 1993;103(5):1336–42.

[135] Rajala R, Partinen M, Sane T, et al. Obstructive sleep apnoea syndrome in morbidly obese patients. J Intern Med 1991;230(2):125–9.

[136] Young T, Palta M, Dempsey J, et al. The occurrence of sleep-disordered breathing among middle-aged adults. N Engl J Med 1993;328(17):1230–5.

[137] Davies RJ, Stradling JR. The relationship between neck circumference, radiographic pharyngeal anatomy, and the obstructive sleep apnoea syndrome. Eur Respir J 1990;3(5): 509–14.

[138] Katz I, Stradling J, Slutsky AS, et al. Do patients with obstructive sleep apnea have thick necks? Am Rev Respir Dis 1990;141(5 Pt 1):1228–31.

[139] Harman EM, Wynne JW, Block AJ. The effect of weight loss on sleep-disordered breathing and oxygen desaturation in morbidly obese men. Chest 1982;82(3):291–4.

[140] Smith PL, Gold AR, Meyers DA, et al. Weight loss in mildly to moderately obese patients with obstructive sleep apnea. Ann Intern Med 1985;103(6 (Pt 1)):850–5.

[141] Suratt PM, McTier RF, Findley LJ, et al. Changes in breathing and the pharynx after weight loss in obstructive sleep apnea. Chest 1987;92(4):631–7.

[142] Wolf AM, Colditz GA. Current estimates of the economic cost of obesity in the United States. Obes Res 1998;6(2):97–106.

[143] Colditz GA. Economic costs of obesity and inactivity. Med Sci Sports Exerc 1999;31(Suppl 11):S663–7.

[144] Seidell JC. The impact of obesity on health status: some implications for health care costs. Int J Obes Relat Metab Disord 1995;19(Suppl 6):S13–6.

[145] Birmingham CL, Muller JL, Palepu A, et al. The cost of obesity in Canada. CMAJ 1999; 160(4):483–8.

[146] Oster G, Thompson D, Edelsberg J, et al. Lifetime health and economic benefits of weight loss among obese persons. Am J Public Health 1999;89(10):1536–42.

ELSEVIER
SAUNDERS

SURGICAL
CLINICS OF
NORTH AMERICA

Surg Clin N Am 85 (2005) 703–723

Dietary and Medical Therapy of Obesity

Phyllis Stumbo, PhD, RD, Donna Hemingway, MS, RD,
William G. Haynes, MBChB, MD*

*General Clinical Research Center, Carver College of Medicine, 200 Hawkins Drive,
University of Iowa, Iowa City, IA 52242, USA*

There has been a dramatic worldwide rise in the prevalence of obesity, which is associated with substantial morbidity and mortality from cardiovascular and other diseases. There are standardized cut-off points for the recommendation of various treatments, beginning conservatively with diet and behavior modification, followed by pharmacotherapy, and, after failure of these treatments, consideration of bariatric surgery. Early in the 1990s, body mass index (BMI; Wt $(kg)/Ht$ $(m)^2$) became the standard unit for classifying weight. Table 1 indicates the most recent classifications published by the World Health Organization [1].

Genetics may dictate to some degree how much danger obesity poses for an individual. For example, according to Seidell and Rissanen [2], people living in South Asia and China and probably Asians living elsewhere have an increased absolute health risk, particularly for type 2 diabetes at all levels of BMI. Some recommend setting a BMI of 23 for overweight and 25 or 27 for obesity in Asian populations [3].

In addition to overall adiposity, greater deposition of abdominal fat (visceral obesity) is associated with alterations in glucose/insulin homeostasis, hypertension, dyslipidemia, and the metabolic syndrome [4,5]. The National Institutes of Health (NIH) publication, *Practical Guide: Identification, Evaluation, and Treatment of Overweight and Obesity in Adults,* links a waist circumference greater than 88 cm in women and 102 in men with increased health risk [6]. These NIH guidelines outline obesity treatment strategies based on the health risks associated with increasing degrees of obesity and the presence of comorbidities. Reduction of food intake, increase in physical activity, and individualized lifestyle strategies are recommended once BMI exceeds 25. The addition of pharmacotherapy is

* Corresponding author.
E-mail address: William-g-haynes@uiowa.edu (W.G. Haynes).

0039-6109/05/$ - see front matter © 2005 Elsevier Inc. All rights reserved.
doi:10.1016/j.suc.2005.04.002   *surgical.theclinics.com*

Table 1
Classification of adults according to body mass index

Classification	BMI (kg/m^2)	Risk of comorbidities
Underweight	Below 18.5	Low (but risk of other clinical problems is increased)
Normal range	18.5–24.9	Average
Overweight	25.0 or higher	
Preobese	25.0–29.9	Increased
Obese class I	30.0–34.9	Moderately increased
Obese class II	35.0–39.9	Severely increased
Obese class III	40 or higher	Very severely increased

Data from World Health Organization. Obesity: preventing and managing the global epidemic. WHO Technical Report Series, No. 894. World Health Organization; 2000.

appropriate when BMI reaches 30 (or at 27 with comorbidities). Bariatric surgery is not recommended until BMI reaches 40 (or 35 with comorbidities) (Table 2).

Comorbidities include coronary artery disease, other atherosclerotic disease, type 2 diabetes, and sleep apnea. Additional cardiovascular risk factors include cigarette smoking, hypertension ($>140/90$ mm Hg), elevated low-density lipoprotein (LDL) cholesterol levels (>130 mg/dL), decreased high-density lipoprotein (HDL) cholesterol levels (<35 mg/dL), impaired fasting glucose (100–125 mg/dL), family history of premature coronary heart disease, and advancing age (≥ 45 years for men and ≥ 55 years for women). Three or more cardiovascular risk factors in an obese patient are assumed to confer the same risk as a comorbidity [6]. Other obesity-related diseases include gynecologic abnormalities, osteoarthritis, gallstones, and stress incontinence, which do not confer increased risk of death but do contribute to morbidity [7].

Principles of dietary treatment for obesity

The cornerstone of dietary obesity treatment is reduced energy intake. The desired outcome of negative energy balance is to lose body fat, spare muscle

Table 2
Recommended obesity treatment strategies for different weight classifications

Classification	BMI (kg/m^2)	Treatment
Overweight	25.0 or higher	Decrease calorie intake Increase activity Counseling strategies to improve quality of life
Preobese	27.0–29.9	Add pharmacotherapy if comorbidities are present
Obese class I	30.0–34.9	Add pharmacotherapy
Obese class II	35.0–39.9	Consider bariatric surgery if comorbidities are present
Obese class III	40 or higher	Consider bariatric surgery

protein, normalize blood lipids, stabilize blood glucose, and reduce hypertension. The low calorie diet (LCD) commonly used by health professionals in clinical programs is outlined in Table 3. The LCD typically is designed to be from 500 to 1000 calories below daily energy needs to produce a weight loss of 1 to 2 pounds (0.5– 1.0 kg) per week. In general, the LCD uses a low-fat component fueled in part by studies of heart disease and diabetes and partly by the higher energy value of fats compared with protein and carbohydrate. Patients with metabolic dyslipidemic syndrome (triglyceride levels >150 or HDL levels <35 mg/dL) may have lipid and cardiovascular benefit from relatively high intake of unsaturated fat (30%–35% of calories). If the weight loss required to achieve a normal BMI is between 5 and 10 kg, this loss can be accomplished within the confines of a 3- to 4- month program. If the excess weight is greater, as with an initial BMI of 35 (25 kg excess weight) or 40 (37 kg excess weight), a longer program is required. Health benefits become evident before optimal weight is reached. Even a modest weight loss of 5% to 10% of body weight can improve glycemic control and blood lipid levels and reduce blood pressure [8].

When the medical risk of continued obesity is extreme, as with obstructive sleep apnea, weight loss can be hastened by developing more stringent dietary plans. A medically supervised very low calorie diet (VLCD) of less than 800 calories (1000–2000 calorie deficit) supplies a minimal amount of energy and enough essential nutrients to avoid side effects (Table 4). A VLCD reduces the time needed to reach a weight goal by one half or

Table 3
Characteristics of the low-calorie diet

Definition	Components
Energy deficit of 500–1000 kcal/day	Considers food likes and dislikes
Daily intake:	Limits fat intake but considers the function and beneficial qualities of different types of fat
1000–1200 calories for women	Encourages ample protein intake from plant sources and lean animal and aquatic sources
1200–1600 calories for men	Encourages ample intakes of fiber from a variety of plant sources including whole grains, vegetables, fruits
	Limits alcohol intake to two drinks per day, if at all
	Gives attention to adequate intake of calcium at 1000–1500 mg/day, particularly from dairy products
	Includes vitamin and mineral supplementation at a level of 100% of the dietary reference intake

Table 4
Characteristics of the very low calorie diet

Definition	Components

Calorie deficit >1000 kcal/day	Is used in limited circumstances
	  by specialized and experienced practitioners
	Is reserved for BMI >30, or after
	  failure of other approaches, or when
	  risk of continued obesity is extreme
	Uses either a liquid protein supplement or
	  protein from meat, fish, or poultry to spare
	  the loss of lean body tissue
	Protein-sparing modified fast includes low-carbohydrate
	  component
	Requires supplemental vitamins and minerals

more. These diets may use liquid formulas or high-protein foods with nutritional supplements. A variation of the VLCD is the protein-sparing modified fast with a carbohydrate restriction to less than 40 g/d. The modern VLCD contains adequate carbohydrate, potassium, magnesium, and other nutrients and minerals and leads to significant weight reduction without the cardiac arrhythmias described with early VLCD diets. Even so, regular evaluation of baseline and follow-up markers of nutritional status (hematocrit, red blood cell indices, liver enzymes, electrolytes) and cardiovascular function (electrocardiograph QTc) of individuals receiving VLCDs are recommended. Unfortunately, the benefit of a significantly higher initial weight loss on the VLCD seems to be short term. Several studies indicate that after 1 to 5 years the weight loss with a VLCD is not significantly different from that with a LCD [9–11].

Diet composition

The consuming public has an avid interest in diet composition, especially as it relates to weight control and weight reduction. Popular weight-reduction diets enjoy a following for a time, fall out of favor, and tend to resurface periodically. Weight-loss diets that limit intake of carbohydrates have increased in popularity dramatically in recent years, and a number of research studies indicate diet composition may play an important role in weight loss and maintenance of weight changes [12]. The success of very low carbohydrate diets is attributed to ketosis and the subsequent loss of appetite that develops from consumption of dietary fats in the absence of carbohydrate, but the bottom line is that self-selected diets devoid of carbohydrate are lower in total energy value [13]. Volek and Sharman [14] summarized their studies investigating the effect of a low carbohydrate diet on metabolic parameters and report numerous metabolic benefits, including reduced serum triglyceride levels, increased HDL levels, decreased total serum cholesterol levels, improvement in LDL particle size, decreased serum insulin levels, increased production of thyroid hormone, decreased total and truncal fat mass, and increased in lean body mass. Of further benefit, weight loss alone reduced inflammatory markers [14].

Layman and associates [15] have studied the effects of a moderate protein/moderate carbohydrate diet on weight loss, body fat loss, muscle-sparing, triglyceride and HDL levels, and stability of blood sugar. A 1700-calorie diet providing 9 to 10 oz high-quality protein (ie, eggs, dairy protein, and muscle proteins from meat, poultry, and fish) and three servings of dairy foods was compared with a standard 1700-calorie low-fat diet. They found that increasing the proportion of protein to carbohydrate from the standard low-fat diet had positive effects on body composition, blood lipid levels, glucose homeostasis, and satiety during weight loss.

Epidemiologic and experimental data suggest dietary calcium plays a role in energy metabolism and weight regulation in humans [16]. Data from animal models present evidence of a role for intracellular calcium in the regulation of lipogenesis and lipolysis [17]. Zemel and associates [18] demonstrated in obese adults that a reduced calorie diet supplemented with 800 mg calcium alone or a high-dairy diet supplying 1200 to 1300 mg calcium from diary foods exerts a beneficial effect compared with a standard diet containing 400 to 500 mg calcium. The results included increased weight loss and a greater percent of fat lost from the trunk region, with diary products exhibiting a substantially greater effect than calcium alone.

These research outcomes should interest clinicians following patients after bariatric surgery. The need for adequate protein and calcium seems to be critical for the metabolic success of patients undergoing weight loss through reduced energy intake.

Increasing energy output

Diet (energy input) is only half of the energy equation; the second half is energy output. The current obesogenic environment includes laborsaving devices and machines that promote inactivity and remove much of the physical effort from activities of daily living [19]. Although increasing activity alone is not enough to promote weight loss, it enhances the success of a LCD [20] and is essential to avoid unwanted weight gain or regain after losing weight [21]. Increasing physical activity is not merely an option for weight loss and weight maintenance—it is an essential component of success and a major lifestyle intervention challenge for physicians, health professionals, and patients alike. The goal is to optimize energy expenditure, maintain metabolically active tissue, and prevent musculoskeletal injuries [22]. Table 5 suggests appropriate ways to increase activity at progressively higher levels of obesity with cautionary use of weight-bearing activities for the profoundly obese. Table 6 lists factors to consider when promoting increased activity or an exercise program with selected patients.

Table 5
Recommended activity and exercise modalities based on Body mass index

Modality	BMI category			
	25–29.9	30–34.9	35–39.9	>40
Reduce time watching television	+	+	+	+
Increase leisure time activity	+	+	+	+
Add non–weight-bearing activity: swimming, cycling, strength/resistance training, arm aerobics, chair aerobics, ergometer, recline bike	+	+	+	+
Alternate weight-bearing with non–weight-bearing activity and interval walking	+	++	++	++
Brisk walking	+	++	++	++
Daily structured weight-bearing activity: exercise class, exercise video, sports, dance	+	++	++	++

+, May be initiated without medical supervision; ++, requires regular medical monitoring.

Individuals with a BMI above 30 or factors increasing the risk of injury, dehydration, or cardiac dysfunction would benefit from careful assessment by a physician and regular monitoring or supervision from a qualified health professional when weight-bearing activities are recommended.

An exercise prescription for an obese individual should entail three stages: initiating the exercise or activity, achieving the optimal level of expenditure for weight reduction, and stressing the on-going effort required for weight maintenance and preventing weight gain [23,24]. Improvement in health risks such as impaired glucose tolerance, hypertension, and dyslipidemia can be achieved with a exercise of lower intensity and duration than required for improved cardiovascular fitness. The level of exercise required to maintain a lower body weight after weight reduction is greater than that required during the energy-restricted phase [24,25]. One simple

Table 6
Factors to consider when beginning an exercise program

Factor	Concern
Age, gender	Men age ≥45 and women ≥55 years at increased relative risk for cardiovascular disease and age related degenerative disease
Years of sedentary lifestyle	Increased risk of injury, dehydration, or cardiac arrest
Presence of asthma, chronic obstructive pulmonary disease, heart disease, joint disease, osteoporosis, recent fractures	Increased risk of injury, dehydration, or cardiac arrest

approach to the need for gradually increasing exercise is to recommend purchase of a pedometer, asking patients to keep written records of daily step counts. Patients can be advised to increase the daily step count by approximately 10% per week. This approach also can be used to assess the patient's compliance with advice, and it encourages discussion of attitudes about exercise and potential limitations. Most activities are more strenuous for obese patients than for those who have lost excess weight. Table 7 describes special considerations and characteristics of these three exercise stages. Care must be taken to avoid sore muscles and the fatigue or injury that can occur when the activity level is increased too rapidly. Injuries must be avoided, or the inactivity imposed during recovering from injury will undermine weight-loss efforts.

Many overweight and obese individuals are challenged by body heat and sweat produced during exercise. Swimming minimizes heat stress and reduces the load on joints. Loose-fitting clothing prevents abrasion, chaffing, and overheating. Applying petroleum jelly to the skin between the thighs and in the armpit area can prevent chafing as well. Although exercise often is difficult to do, the benefits go beyond the energy cost. Exercise reduces negative mood [26,27,28] and is associated with improved sleep quality [29,30].

Table 7
Activity prescription by treatment stage

Goal: activity level	Considerations and benefits
Initiating activity level: 30 min/day or 150 min/week (5 days, 30 min/day)	Provides beneficial effects on cardiovascular disease and diabetes
	Supports the low-calorie diet and enhances weight loss efforts
	Insufficient to provide maintenance of lost weight
	May be in the form of intermittent bouts of exercise lasting 10–15 minutes
Activity level to promote weight loss: 40–60 min/day or 200–300 min/week	Often presents a significant challenge to achieve
	Results in significant improvement in cardiovascular health
	May decrease negative mood
	Intensity of workout does not effect body weight or composition as much as total time spent in the activity
Activity level to maintain lost weight and avoid weight gain: 60 min/day or 300 min/week	Required for long-term maintenance of weight loss
	Commonly includes activities such as walking, cycling, weight lifting, aerobics, running, stair climbing
	May be more successful when the activity can be done at or from home

Pharmacotherapy for obesity

In general, pharmacotherapy is indicated for patients who have a BMI more than 30 without comorbidities or more than 27 with at least one comorbidity (or three or more cardiovascular risk factors) (see Table 2). Persons who achieve a weight loss of more than 0.5 kg/wk in the first month of pharmacotherapy are more likely to have a sustained and substantial response to longer-term treatment. This information can be used to optimize treatment and prevent excessive cost. Most existing agents have not been rigorously tested in combination with other weight-reducing agents, although combination therapy often is used to achieve clinically significant weight loss.

Therapies currently approved for weight loss by the Food and Drug Administration include orlistat and sibutramine. Orlistat is a nonabsorbed intestinal lipase inhibitor that reduces dietary fat absorption by about 30% at a dose of 120 mg three times each day. Randomized trials have shown that patients receiving orlistat have a weight loss of about 10% over a 12-month period, compared with a 5% weight reduction with placebo [31,32]. Weight loss is sustained for at least 4 years with continued therapy [Orlistat Prescribing Information, US.gsk.com/products/assets/us_advandamet.pdf. Accessed March 2005]. In addition to inducing weight loss, orlistat lowers LDL levels by about 6%, although this reduction is not accompanied by an increase in HDL cholesterol levels [31,32]. These lipid changes presumably reflect weight loss and decreased absorption of saturated and unsaturated fats. Orlistat also reduces the risk of developing diabetes by about two thirds in at-risk obese subjects [33] and lowers glycosylated hemoglobin levels by about 0.5% in obese patients who have type 2 diabetes [34]. In a substantial minority of patients who continue to eat significant amounts of dietary fat, orlistat causes gastrointestinal symptoms (fecal urgency, incontinence, or anal leakage) related to the presence of unabsorbed fat in the colon and stool. One disadvantage of orlistat is that it must be taken three times a day, with the potential that patients selectively miss doses when they desire a high-fat meal.

Sharma and Golay [35] have documented that patients treated with orlistat lose more weight and have greater decreases in blood pressure than patients treated with placebo. Compared with lifestyle interventions alone, systolic pressure is reduced by about 5 mm Hg and diastolic pressure by about 2 mm Hg. A reduction in blood pressure of this magnitude by antihypertensive therapy would be expected to reduce major cardiovascular events by 10% to 20%, so this effect is potentially important [36]. For a given weight loss, however, the reduction in blood pressure is no greater in patients treated with orlistat than in patients who lose weight with diet alone. There is thus no evidence that orlistat lowers blood pressure except by promoting weight loss. These beneficial hypotensive effects of orlistat-induced weight loss contrast with the effects on blood pressure of the other major drug that is licensed for weight loss, sibutramine.

Sibutramine blocks norepinephrine, serotonin, and dopamine reuptake in the central nervous system. Sibutramine, at a dose of 15 mg/d, causes a placebo-corrected 5% long-term weight loss, similar to that observed with orlistat, with studies lasting up to 2 years [37]. Sibutramine seems to have particularly pronounced effects on preventing weight regain, with the difference between placebo and sibutramine being 4 kg at 1 year and 7 kg at 2 years [38]. Patients who fail to lose 2 kg during the first month of sibutramine treatment are unlikely to achieve a weight loss greater than 5% by 6 months; only 20% of these patients lost more than 2 kg [Sibutramine Prescribing Information, March 2005]. In addition, after an initial 4-week period of sibutramine therapy, intermittent use of sibutramine (12 weeks on drug, 6 weeks off drug) seems to be as effective in reducing weight (−8.1% average loss) as continuous use (−8.2% average loss) over 48 weeks [37]. Sibutramine has been shown to be effective in reducing weight in patients already taking metformin, with an additional 6-kg average weight loss after 12 months [39]. Sibutramine does not decrease LDL levels but does increase HDL levels by about 4%, in contrast to orlistat [37]. Sibutramine reduces glycosylated hemoglobin by about 0.5% in obese diabetic patients [40]. Despite weight loss, sibutramine does not decrease arterial pressure [37], however, and some obese hypertensive patients develop marked hypertension while taking sibutramine. Headache, dry mouth, and constipation occur in about 10% of patients treated with sibutramine [37].

Several drugs approved for other indications also cause weight loss. These agents may be particularly useful for patients whose insurers will not pay for specific antiobesity drugs. One such agent is the insulin-sensitizing and antihyperglycemic drug metformin, which has been used in nondiabetic obese patients to induce weight losses of about 3% to 5% [41]. This weight loss is accompanied by decreases in LDL and insulin levels, without hypoglycemia, even at doses of 850 mg, three times each day. The antidepressant and smoking-cessation agent bupropion inhibits norepinephrine and dopamine reuptake. Treatment with bupropion at doses of 200 to 400 mg/d decreased weight by 5% to 13% in randomized clinical trials [42,43]. The antiepileptic medication topiramate can also cause weight loss (∼8% greater than diet alone with dosages of 200–300 mg/d). Weight loss after topiramate treatment is associated with improvements in blood pressure and glucose tolerance [44].

Dietary management of obesity surgery patients

Nutrition is a critical aspect of obesity treatment. Patients exploring bariatric surgery options should have attempted the previously discussed conservative methods of treatment without success at least twice over a period of at least 2 years before surgery is considered appropriate. Gastric reduction or bypass procedure is considered successful when the permanently reduced energy intake results in at least a 50% reduction in body weight and symptoms of the comorbidities of diabetes, coronary heart disease, and sleep apnea are improved or resolved. Because the surgery is designed to produce a state of semi-starvation, careful evaluation and monitoring are required preoperatively, postoperatively, and at annual follow-ups to improve outcomes and avoid serious malnutrition and other complications.

Physical, social, and psychological assessments are part of the presurgery evaluation. Patient compliance with scheduled follow-up visits for monitoring cardiovascular and nutritional parameters is necessary to avoid potentially life-threatening complications. The patient must hold a realistic view of the lifelong care and attention required for a successful outcome. The clinical interview, at least 3 months before surgery, should [45]:

Evaluate previous weight loss attempts and treatments to ensure each surgical patient has failed conventional therapy.

Evaluate eating patterns, eating disorder symptoms, physical activity, and attitudes and expectations for the surgical treatment to prepare properly for follow-up after surgery.

Assess psychiatric history and mental and marital status to prepare for the ancillary support required for the long recovery period expected after bariatric surgery.

No single psychologic pattern fits all obese patients, but general characteristics have been described. Morbidly obese persons often exhibit patterns of compulsive eating, which may include binge eating disorder (rapid ingestion of large amounts of food, with a feeling of loss of control and subsequent guilt and self-condemnation) or grazing (eating smaller amounts of food continuously throughout the day). Others suggest that surgical candidates report noncompulsive eating, such as mindless eating, and frequent snacking on high-calorie foods and beverages. Studies suggest that one third to one half of patients seeking treatment for obesity suffer from binge eating disorder. It is fairly common for patients to report that they have lost touch with how much they need to eat to feel full and that they look forward to "learning how to eat again" after surgery [46].

A nutritionist's involvement is important to help patients understand their current eating patterns, assess the nutritional quality of their intake, and identify changes required after surgery to minimize food volume and carbohydrate content. Researchers have attempted to match the surgical method to preoperative eating habits. Sugarman and colleagues [47] blame the abuse of sweets in preference to more nutritious solid food for inconsistent weight loss after vertical-banded gastroplasty (VBG). Brolin and colleagues [48] undertook a prospective study to determine if preoperative evaluation of eating could predict satisfactory weight loss after VGB surgery. They suggested that patients who ate large quantities of food at regular intervals (mealtimes) were the best candidates for VGB, and grazers were the poorest candidates. Roux-en-Y gastric bypass was recommended for sweet-eaters or snackers. After surgery, a substantial number of patients who underwent VBG became sweet- and ice cream-eaters because they could not comfortably consume even small quantities of meat, vegetables, and fruit [48]. These findings reinforce the need for close dietary evaluation and monitoring.

Nutritional recommendations during the presurgery phase are to maximize protein intake and correct suboptimal nutritional parameters such as below-normal hemoglobin. Patients begin supplementing intake with a reliable source of vitamin B_{12}, protein, and a broad-spectrum multivitamin/mineral at 100% recommended dietary allowance/adequate intake (Table 8). Andersen and Larsen [49] found that despite thorough instruction, close follow-up, and the appropriate surgical procedure, quality of diet did not improve in 18 patients followed for 2 years [49]. Major nutrient insufficiencies can be anticipated and prevented with supplementation. Even so, patients are expected to begin a nutrient-dense hypocaloric diet in the short term to reduce body weight by 1% to 2% as appropriate training for surgery. Writing a sample postsurgery diet is a good way to give the patient a realistic picture of life after surgery. Some clinics require the patient to demonstrate the ability to record a 3-day food plan for eating at home as if the surgery had been performed. If the plan is not completed, the clinic visit is cancelled. Patients must also demonstrate the ability to increase activity level in preparation for adopting a healthier life style after surgery.

Dietary guidelines after gastric surgery vary depending on the type of surgery and the practices and experiences of the surgical staff but generally involve attention to fluid intake, food consistency, food volume, and overall dietary adequacy:

Meals should consist of small quantities of food and be pureed, soft, or easily chewed.

Meals need to last 20 minutes or more to avoid bolus eating and to allow satiety to occur.

High-protein foods should be eaten preferentially at meals.

To avoid protein malnutrition, 60 g protein is recommended daily.

Liquids should be ingested well before meals or at least 30 minutes afterwards.

Foods that are dry (roast beef, turkey), sticky (peanut butter), gummy (fresh bread), or stringy (celery, fibrous fruit and vegetables) present the biggest problems.

There are also nutritional concerns in the months following the surgery [50].

Gastric-restriction procedures may produce iron and vitamin B_{12} deficiencies.

Gastric restriction with bypass (Roux-en-Y) procedure can cause nutrient deficiencies of iron, vitamin B_{12}, calcium, and folic acid. In addition,

Table 8
Recommended nutrient allowances for men and women age 14–70 years in the United States

Age group (years)	Protein (g)	Vitamin A (g)	Vitamin D (μg)	Vitamin E (mg)	Vitamin K (μg)	Thiamin (g)	Ribo flavin (g)	Niacin (g)	Folate (μg)	Vitamin B_{12} (μg)	Panto-thenate (mg)	Biotin (μg)	Choline (mg)
Men
14-18	52	900	5	15	75	1.2	1.3	16	400	2.4	5	25	550
19-50	56	900	5	15	120	1.2	1.3	16	400	2.4	5	30	550
51-70	56	900	10	15	120	1.2	1.3	16	400	2.4	5	30	550
Women
14-18	34	700	5	15	75	1.0	1.0	14	400	2.4	5	25	400
19-50	46	700	5	15	90	1.1	1.1	14	400	2.4	5	30	425
51-70	46	700	10	15	90	1.1	1.1	14	400	2.4	5	30	425

Age group (years)	Calcium (mg)	Chromium (μg)	Copper (μg)	Fluoride (μg)	Iodine (μg)	Iron (mg)	Magnesium (mg)	Manganese (mg)	Molybdenum (μg)	Phosphorus (mg)	Selenium (μg)	Zinc (mg)	N-3 fatty acid (g)
Men
14-18	1300	35	890	3	150	11	410	2.2	43	1250	55	11	1.7
19-50	1000	35	900	4	150	8	400-20	2.3	45	700	55	11	1.6
51-70	1200	30	900	4	150	8	420	2.3	45	700	55	11	1.6
Women
14-18	1300	24	890	3	150	15	360	1.6	43	1250	55	9	1.1
19-50	1000	25	900	3	150	18	310-20	1.8	45	700	55	8	1.1
51-70	1200	20	900	3	150	8	320	1.8	45	700	55	8	1.1

Recommended dietary allowances (RDA) where available and adequate intake (AI) for nutrients without an RDA.
Data from Trumbo P, Schlicker S, Yates AA, et al. Dietary reference intakes for energy, carbohydrate, fiber, fat, fatty acids, cholesterol, protein and amino acids. J Am Dietet Assoc 2002;102:1623–5.

dumping syndrome (diarrhea following concentrated carbohydrate intake) is common with this procedure.
Biliopancreatic diversion procedures have even greater risk for nutrient deficiencies.
Fat malabsorption and lactose intolerance can cause concerns in patients who have undergone biliopancreatic diversion.
Dehydration and gallstone formation are concerns for all bariatric surgical procedures.
A vitamin/mineral supplement is highly recommended.

The period of weight loss before surgery should be monitored by the physician to ensure the patient is sufficiently nourished to heal normally after surgery and is psychologically prepared for the realities of self-care and relinquishing some of the pleasures of eating. Nutritional recommendations before surgery include inclusion of a minimum of 60 g protein/d and adequate fruits, vegetables, and dairy products to provide the recommended dietary allowances of vitamins and minerals (Table 8) [51]. This training is important to ensure the patient is nutritionally replete and will heal properly after surgery and to train the patient in developing a nutritionally adequate diet after surgery.

Careful compliance with a prescribed diet after surgery is essential to ensure weight loss and protect the newly formed stomach pouch and intestinal graft. Table 9 outlines a typical dietary prescription after surgery. The diet is liquid-only (water or clear liquids) for the first day or two, with progression in a few days to a pureed or blended diet and gradual liberalization of diet. By 1 month after surgery, the diet includes normal foods, although the need to limit food selections may be more or less permanent. Problem foods are poorly chewed steaks and chops, apple skins, citrus fruit membranes, incompletely chewed raw or fibrous vegetables, and fresh bread (because of the tendency to form a solid "bread ball" in the stomach pouch; toasting prevents this problem).

Gastric-restriction procedures can produce marked malnutrition that, when left untreated, may lead to a starvation syndrome that can result to death or permanent disability. The risk for this condition is particularly high when the gastric pouch or outlet is too small after surgery or when persistent uncontrolled eating leads to repeated vomiting. Patients may react to repeated vomiting by limiting intake to liquids, resulting in inadequate nutrient intake and eventual malnutrition. Mason [52] cautions gastric surgeons to be alert for symptoms of protein malnutrition, refeeding syndrome, and Wernicke–Korsakoff syndrome. Protein malnutrition is marked by a low serum albumin level and can occur when body weight is normal. Wasting is easy to recognize in a thin person, but marked obesity can mask the loss of muscle mass. Refeeding syndrome is characterized by a drop in serum phosphorus level during rapid refeeding that cannot be corrected by addition of phosphate to the refeeding solution. Proper treatment is gradual

Table 9
Dietary progression from clear liquids to solid food following bariatric surgery

Time[a] (days)	Description	Example–food (grams of protein per serving)
1–3	Clear liquid	Six meals: 1 oz broth (0.1–0.6 g) 1 oz. high protein fruit drink (1.1 g) (Total protein intake = 8–10 g/d)
2–28	Blended diet	Breakfast: 1 oz yogurt (1.2 g) 2 oz liquid supplement[b] (4.0 g) Lunch 1 oz cream soup[c] (1.7 g) 1 oz pudding (0.6 g) 1 oz liquid supplement[b] (2.0 g) Dinner 1 oz cream soup[c] (1.7 g) 1 oz yogurt (1.2 g) 1 oz liquid supplement[b] (2.0 g) Snacks (×3) 8 oz instant breakfast (16 g × 3 snacks) (Total protein intake = 62.4 g/d)
7–28	Transition to solid food— add 1 oz of one new soft food every 2–3 days at meals (no more than 6 oz total per meal)	After 1 week: Scrambled eggs[d], cottage cheese[c,d], low-fat refried beans, crackers, mashed potatoes[c], cream of wheat[c], dry cereal with milk After 3 weeks: tuna salad[d], ground chicken or turkey[d], baked fish[d], canned vegetables, banana, watermelon or cantaloupe (no seeds)
	Other rules:	Sip at least 6 cups water or low-calorie beverage during the day in addition to meals

[a] Time at each stage varies.
[b] Liquid supplements are high-protein, low-sugar beverages such as Sugar-Free Carnation Breakfast (Glendale, California), Atkins shakes (Ronkonkoma, New York), or milk with added skim milk powder. High-protein fruit drinks are commercially available fruit drinks containing whey or egg white protein.
[c] Cottage cheese and any food with particles larger than a pea should be blended. Add 1 one-third cup dry skim milk powder/cup of food or milk to increase protein content.
[d] These foods add 3–6 g protein/oz.

refeeding. Patients who have undergone gastric-reduction surgery and who are not taking a multivitamin containing thiamine are at risk for Wernicke–Korsakoff syndrome, which is characterized by peripheral and central nervous system damage that may occur 2 to 3 months after the onset of persistent vomiting. A vitamin supplement that contains thiamine is the best insurance against this condition. The condition of the gut as a whole is a critical component in facilitating adequate nutrient absorption [53].

Counseling techniques to improve treatment outcome

A complete approach to every obesity treatment includes focus on lifestyle change supporting the patient's treatment plan. Weight loss and maintenance of a lower body weight seem be natural for some and impossible for others and have been extensively studied [54–57]. Weight-loss interventions with the greatest intensity tend to produce the greatest weight loss. Long-term success seems to depend on continuing the lifestyle changes learned during intensive interventions, namely high levels of physical activity and continued monitoring of body weight and food intake [20]. Many studies have asked why people overeat and become overfat [58,59], but, whatever the reason for the overweight, obese people need training and continued encouragement to adjust intake appropriately, exercise adequately, and maintain health-promoting behaviors.

Weight-control counselors use a variety of techniques to support the level of motivation needed to change behavior and incorporate rewards for continuing new behaviors (Table 10). When individually applied, these counseling techniques have the potential to improve outcomes of obesity treatment at all levels, from basic, diet-only programs to extensive interventions including bariatric surgery.

Techniques vary in their focus. Motivational interviewing is patient-focused and uses empathy and acceptance to identify, explore, and resolve the ambivalence the patient expresses toward behavior change. The interview is designed to elicit patient participation rather than provide clinician dominance. Sensitivity to the patient's readiness to make a change is a salient part of the process. It is most effective when used at the beginning of the weight loss effort. Motivational interviewing as part of a weight loss program may overlap with cognitive behavioral training [60–64].

Behavioral approaches use knowledge from record-keeping, support of environmental change, visualizations, and reward systems. Behavioral techniques include teaching new skills, problem solving, goal setting, establishing social support, and stimulus control. Persons reporting successful long-term weight loss continue to self-monitor their eating and exercise behaviors. Long- term studies indicate support for these techniques must be sustained for the new behaviors to be continued [65,66].

Training in self-nurturing and limit-setting skills is the basis for the solution method. Research has shown that when people master the skills of nurturing and setting limits from within, they feel balanced, happy, and secure, and the drive to soothe and comfort themselves with food ends. These skills are taught through coaching and group participation. The skills are used consciously at first but become spontaneous after 12 to 18 months as neural networks in the brain are rewired. This training program is intensive and is limited currently by the number of trained providers. It shows promise for eliciting neurobiologic changes similar to drug therapies designed to turn off the drive to overeat [67].

Summary

Surgery is not a cure for obesity but is an effective tool for limiting food consumption. If severely obese patients do not respond to a treatment plan

Table 10
Description and techniques used in several counseling techniques

Technique	Description	Techniques
Motivational interviewing	A directive, client-centered counseling style for eliciting behavior change by helping clients explore and resolve ambivalence	Is focused and goal oriented
		Therapist expresses empathy and acceptance
		Is shaped by the therapist's understanding of triggers for change
		May overlap with cognitive behavioral training
		Supports self-directed changes
Behavioral approach	A functional analysis of behavior, delineating the association between eating and exercise behaviors and environmental events	Self-monitoring is the centerpiece
		Targets food choices, time of day, mood, eating style, presence of other people, other activities, and physical activity
		Uses positive reinforcement systems to encourage change
		Teaches specific skills (eg, low-fat diet, portion control, exercise)
		Techniques include stimulus control, problem solving, cognitive restructuring, relapse prevention
		Long-term effectiveness requires continued support
Developmental skills training (the solution method)	A training program that supports homeostasis and integrates understandings and methods from developmental psychology, family systems, biomedical, genetic, neurobiology and behavioral theories of the etiology of obesity	Focuses on mastery of developmental skills (nurturing and limit-setting) and mastery living (balanced eating, regular exercise, health maintenance, body acceptance, meaningful pursuits, and time to restore)

Table 10 (*continued*)

Technique	Description	Techniques
Developmental skills training (the solution method)		Skills are used consciously at first; with long-term training (18 months or more), skills become spontaneous as neural networks in the brain are rewired and psychosocial development is facilitated Emphasizes a decrease in excessive appetites for food and other common excesses rather than a forced behavior change Is provided by trained healthcare professionals May result in long-term maintenance of beneficial effects Requires active participation for 18 months or longer for skills to become integrated and spontaneous.

that includes nutritional, exercise, and behavioral interventions plus antiobesity drugs, bariatric surgery may be appropriate. When properly selected, the reduced energy value of the limited postsurgery diet can lead to a normal weight for obese patients. In a 10-year follow-up, surgical patients had lost a mean of 16% of presurgery weight, whereas a control group gained 1.6% of body weight [68]. Proper diet selection is important after bariatric surgery and involves more than consideration of the energy value and macronutrient composition. Adequate vitamin and mineral intake is essential to ensure that surgery improves nutritional status. Malabsorption is secondary to some bariatric surgeries and present to some extent with most. Therefore, diet after surgery should be monitored closely for adequacy by a nutritionist.

Acknowledgments

The authors thank Nancy Kraft, RD, LD, University of Iowa Health Care, Iowa City, IA, and Maryann Ludlow, RD, CD, CDE, Fletcher Allen Health Care, Burlington, VT, for their contributions to the discussion of nutrition-counseling practices when preparing for and following bariatric surgery.

References

[1] World Health Organization, Geneva, Switzerland. Obesity: preventing and managing the global epidemic. WHO Technical Report Series, No. 894. World Health Organization; 2000.

[2] Seidell JC, Rissanen AM. Prevalence of obesity in adults: the global epidemic. In: Bray GA, Bouchard C, editors. Handbook of obesity: etiology and pathophysiology. New York: Marcel Dekker; 2004. p. 93–107.

[3] Seidell JC. Obesity insulin resistance and diabetes—a world-wide epidemic. Br J Nutr 2000; 83(Suppl 1):S5–8.

[4] Smith SR, Lovejoy JC, Greenway F, et al. Contributions of total body fat, abdominal subcutaneous adipose tissue compartments, and visceral adipose tissue to the metabolic complications of obesity. Metabolism 2001;50(4):425–35.

[5] Janssen I, Katzmarzyk PT, Ross R. Waist circumference and not body mass index explains obesity-related health risk. Am J Clin Nutr 2004;79:379–84.

[6] National Institutes of Health, Bethesda, Maryland. National Heart, Lung, Bethesda, Maryland, and Blood Institute, North American Association for the Study of Obesity, Silver Springs, Maryland. The practical guide: identification, evaluation, and treatment of overweight and obesity in adults. NIH publication #02–4084.2000. p. 25.

[7] US Department of Health and Human Services. The Surgeon General's call to action to prevent and decrease overweight and obesity. Rockville, MD: US Department of Health and Human Services, Public Health Services, Office of the Surgeon General; 2001.

[8] Goldstein DJ. Beneficial health effects of modest weight loss. Int J Obes Relat Metab Disord 1992;16(6):397–415.

[9] Wadden TA, Foster GD, Letizia KA. One year behavioral treatment of obesity: comparison of moderated and severe calorie restriction and the effects of weight maintenance therapy. J Consult Clin Pschol 1994;62:165–71.

[10] Wing RR, Marcus MD, Salata R, et al. Effects of a very-low-calorie diet on long-term glycemic control in obese type 2 diabetic subjects. Arch Intern Med 1991;151: 1334–40.

[11] Paisey RB, Frost J, Harvey A, et al. Five year results of a prospective very low calorie or conventional weight loss programme in type 2 diabetes. J Hum Nutr Diet 2002;15:121–7.

[12] Halton TL, Hu FB. The effects of high protein diets on thermogenesis, satiety and weight loss: a critical review. J Am Coll Nutr 2004;5:373–85.

[13] Boden G, Sargrad K, Homko C, et al. Effect of a low-carbohydrate diet on appetite, blood glucose levels, and insulin resistance in obese patients with type 2 diabetes. Ann Intern Med 2005;142(6):403–11.

[14] Volek JS, Sharman MJ. Cardiovascular and hormonal aspects of very-low-carbohydrate ketogenic diets. Obes Res 2004;12:115S–23S.

[15] Layman DK, Boileau RA, Erickson DJ, et al. A reduced ratio of dietary carbohydrate to protein improves body composition and blood lipid profiles during weight loss in adult women. J Nutr 2003;133(2):411–7.

[16] Parikh J, Yanovski J. Calcium intake and adiposity. Am J Clin Nutr 2003;77:281–7.

[17] Zemel MB. Role of calcium and diary products in energy partitioning and weight management. Am J Clin Nutr 2004;79(5):907S–12S.

[18] Zemel MB, Thompson W, Milstead A, et al. Calcium and diary acceleration of weight and fat loss during energy restriction in obese adults. Obes Res 2004;12(4):582–90.

[19] Swinburn B, Egger G. Preventive strategies against weight gain and obesity. Obes Rev 2002; 3(4):289–301.

[20] Pavlou KN, Krey S, Steffee WP. Exercise as an adjunct to weight loss and maintenance in moderately obese subjects. Am J Clin Nutr 1989;49:115–23.

[21] Wing RR, Hill JO. Successful weight loss maintenance. Annu Rev Nutr 2001;21:323–41.

[22] Hills AP, Byrne NM. Physical activity in the management of obesity. Clin Dermatol 2004;22: 315–8.

[23] Jakicic JM, Clark K, Coleman E, et al. American College of Sports Medicine position stand. Appropriate intervention strategies for weight loss and the prevention of weight regain in adults. Med Sci Sports Exerc 2001;33(12):2145–56.

[24] Jakicic JM, Winters C, Lang W, et al. Effects of intermittent exercise and use of home exercise equipment on adherence, weight loss, and fitness in overweight women: a randomized trial. JAMA 1999;282(16):1554–60.

[25] van Baak MA, van Mil E, Astrup A, et al. Leisure-time activity is an important determinant of long-term weight maintenance after weight loss in the Sibutramine Trial on Obesity Reduction and Maintenance (STORM trial). Am J Clin Nutr 2003;78:209–14.

[26] Fossati M, Amati F, Painot D, et al. Cognitive behavioral therapy with simultaneous nutritional and physical activity education in obese patients with binge eating disorder. Eat Weight Disord 2004;9(2):134–8.

[27] Lluch A, Hubert P, King NA, et al. Selective effects of acute exercise and breakfast interventions on mood and motivation to eat. Physiol Behav 2000;68(4):515–20.

[28] Thayer RE, Newman JR, McClain TM. Self-regulation of mood: strategies for changing a bad mood, raising energy, and reducing tension. J Pers Soc Psychol 1994;67(5):910–25.

[29] Peppard PE, Young T. Exercise and sleep-disordered breathing: an association independent of body habitus. Sleep 2004;27(3):480–4.

[30] Tanaka H, Shirakawa S. Sleep health, lifestyle, and mental health in the Japanese elderly: ensuring sleep to promote a healthy brain and mind. J Psychosom Res 2004; 56(5):465–77.

[31] Sjöström L, Rissanen A, Andersen T, et al, for the European Multicenter Orlistat Study Group. Randomised placebo-controlled trial of orlistat for weight loss and prevention of weight regain in obese patients. Lancet 1998;352:167–72.

[32] Davidson MH, Hauptman J, DiGirolama M, et al. Weight control and risk factor reduction in obese subjects treated for 2 years with orlistat. A randomized controlled trial. JAMA 1999; 281:235–42.

[33] Heymsfield SB, Segal KR, Hauptman J, et al. Effects of weight loss with orlistat on glucose tolerance and progression to type 2 diabetes in obese adults. Arch Intern Med 2000;160: 1321–6.

[34] Hollander PA, Elbein SC, Hirsch IB, et al. Role of orlistat in the treatment of obese patients with type 2 diabetes. A 1-year randomized double-blind study. Diabetes Care 1998;21: 1288–94.

[35] Sharma AM, Golay A. Effect of orlistat-induced weight loss on blood pressure and heart rate in obese patients with hypertension. J Hypertens 2002;20(9):1873–8.

[36] Collins R, Peto R, MacMahon S, et al. Blood pressure, stroke, and coronary heart disease. Part 2, short-term reductions in blood pressure: overview of randomised drug trials in their epidemiological context. Lancet 1990;335:827–38.

[37] Wirth A, Krause J. Long-term weight loss with sibutramine: a randomized controlled trial. JAMA 2001;286:1331–9.

[38] James WPT, Astrup A, Finer N, et al. Effect of sibutramine on weight maintenance after weight loss: a randomized trial. Lancet 2000;356:2119–25.

[39] McNulty SJ, Ur E, Williams G. Multicenter Sibutramine Study Group. A randomized trial of sibutramine in the management of obese type 2 diabetic patients treated with metformin. Diabetes Care 2003;26(1):125–31.

[40] Fujioka K, Seaton TB, Rowe E, et al, for the Sibutramine/Diabetes Clinical Study Group. Weight loss with sibutramine improves glycaemic control and other metabolic parameters in obese patients with type 2 diabetes mellitus. Diabetes Obes Metab 2000;2:175–87.

[41] Fontbonne A, Charles MA, Juhan-Vague I, et al. The effect of metformin on the metabolic abnormalities associated with upper-body fat distribution. BIGPRO Study Group. Diabetes Care 1996;19:920–6.

[42] Gadde KM, Parker CB, Maner LG, et al. Bupropion for weight loss: an investigation of efficacy and tolerability in overweight and obese women. Obes Res 2001;9:544–51.

[43] Anderson JW, Greenway FL, Fujioka K, et al. Bupropion SR enhances weight loss: a 48 week double-blind, placebo-controlled, trial. Obes Res 2002;10:633–41.

[44] Wilding J, Van Gaal L, Rissanen A, et al, for the OBES-002 Study Group. A randomized double-blind placebo-controlled study of the long-term efficacy and safety of topiramate in the treatment of obese subjects. Int J Obes Relat Metab Disord 2004;28:1399–410.

[45] Sauerland S, Angrisani L, Belachew M, et al. Obesity surgery: evidence-based guidelines of the European Association for Endoscopic Surgery (EAES). Presented at the 12th International Congress of the EAES. Barcelona, Spain, June 2004. Surg Endosc 2005;19(2):200–21.

[46] von Hout GCM, van Oudheusden I, van Heck GL. Psychological profile of the morbidly obese. Obes Surg 2004;14:579–88.

[47] Sugarman HJ, Starkey J, Birkenhauer R. A randomized prospective trial of gastric bypass versus vertical banded gastroplasty for morbid obesity and their effects on sweets versus non-sweets eaters. Ann Surg 1987;205:613–24.

[48] Brolin RE, Robertson LB, Kenler HA, et al. Weight loss and dietary intake after vertical banded gastroplasty and Roux-enY gastric bypass. Ann Surg 1994;220(6):782–90.

[49] Andersen T, Larsen U. Dietary outcome in obese patients treated with a gastroplasty program. Am J Clin Nutr 1989;50:1328–40.

[50] Marcason W. What are the dietary guidelines following bariatric surgery? J Am Dietet Assoc 2004;104:487–8.

[51] Trumbo P, Schlicker S, Yates AA, et al. Dietary reference intakes for energy, carbohydrate, fiber, fat, fatty acids, cholesterol, protein and amino acids. J Am Dietet Assoc 2002;102: 1621–30.

[52] Mason EE. Starvation injury after gastric reduction for obesity. World J Surg 1998;22(9): 1002–7.

[53] Cannizzo F, Kral JG. Obesity surgery: a model of programmed undernutrition. Curr Opin Clin Nutr Metab Care 1998;1(4):363–8.

[54] Flatt JP. What do we most need to learn about food intake regulation? Obes Res 1998;6(4): 307–10.

[55] Astrup A. Dietary composition, substrate balances and body fat in subjects with a predisposition to obesity. Int J Obes Relat Metab Disord 1993;17(3):S32–6; S41–2.

[56] Schrauwen P, Westerterp KR. The role of high-fat diets and physical activity in the regulation of body weight. Br J Nutr 2000;84(4):417–27.

[57] Hill JO, Melanson EL, Wyatt HT. Dietary fat intake and regulation of energy balance: implications for obesity. J Nutr 2000;130(2S Suppl):284S–8S.

[58] Macdiarmid JI, Vail A, Cade JE, et al. The sugar-fat relationship revisited: differences in consumption between men and women of varying BMI. Int J Obes Relat Metab Disord 1998; 22(11):1053–61.

[59] Astrup A, Ryan L, Grunwald GK, et al. The role of dietary fat in body fatness: evidence from a preliminary meta-analysis of ad libitum low-fat dietary intervention studies. Br J Nutr 2000;83:S25–32.

[60] Goldberg JH, Kiernan M. Innovative techniques to address retention in a behavioral weight-loss trial. Health Educ Res 2004, in press.

[61] Rollnick S, Miller WR. What is motivational interviewing? Behav Cogn Psychother 1995;23: 325–34.

[62] Stott NC, Rees M, Rollnick S, et al. Professional responses to innovation in clinical method: diabetes care and negotiating skills. Patient Educ Couns 1996;29(1):67–73.

[63] Wilson TG, Schlam TR. The transtheoretical model and motivational interviewing in the treatment of eating and weight disorders. Clin Psychol Rev 2004;24:361–78.

[64] Smith DE, Heckemeyer CM, Kratt PP, et al. Motivational interviewing to improve adherence to a behavioral weight-control program for older obese women with NIDDM. A pilot study. Diabetes Care 1997;20:52–4.

[65] Wing RR. Behavioral approaches to the treatment of obesity. In: Bray GA, Bouchard C, James WPT, editors. Handbook of obesity. New York: Marcel Dekker; 1998. p. 855–73.

[66] Boutelle KN, Kirschenbaum DS. Further support for consistent self-monitoring as a vital component of successful weight control. Obes Res 1998;6(3):219–24.

[67] Mellin L, Croughan-Minihane M, Dickey L. The solution method: 2 year trends in weight, blood pressure, exercise, depression, and functioning of adults trained in development skills. J Am Diet Assoc 1997;97:1133–8.

[68] Sjostrom L, Lindroos A-K, Peltonen M, et al. Lifestyle, diabetes, and cardiovascular risk factors 10 years after bariatric surgery. N Engl J Med 2004;351(26):2683–93.

ELSEVIER
SAUNDERS

SURGICAL
CLINICS OF
NORTH AMERICA

Surg Clin N Am 85 (2005) 725–740

Patient Selection and the Physiology of Gastrointestinal Antiobesity Operations

Erik Näslund, MD, PhD[a], John G. Kral, MD, PhD[b],*

[a]Division of Surgery, Karolinska Institutet, Danderyd Hospital, SE 182 88 Stockholm, Sweden
[b]Department of Surgery, State University of New York Downstate Medical Center,
Box 40, Brooklyn, NY 11203, USA

Patients who undergo antiobesity surgery pose special problems with regard to preoperative selection because the pathophysiology of obesity influences anesthesia, performance of the surgery, and postoperative care. In addition, to a great extent, the long-term outcomes of antiobesity surgery—positive as well as negative—are independent of the technical performance of the operation. Long-term outcome is important in many types of surgery, but the outcome of antiobesity surgery commonly is judged over longer periods of time and by different standards than other surgery.

Behavioral maladaptation and inability to change detrimental lifestyle factors do not influence most other forms of surgery; notable exceptions are drinking after portal decompression and smoking after coronary bypass surgery. The American College of Surgeons' Statement on Principles Underlying Perioperative Responsibility states: "The surgeon is responsible for the preoperative preparation of the patient. Minimizing the risk of operation while providing maximal opportunity for a satisfactory outcome, requires full appreciation by the surgeon" [1]. In which way does this pertain to patient selection for antiobesity surgery? Optimal outcome has not been well-defined in surgical trials, in general, and in antiobesity surgery, in particular. There are only limited data on patient selection in this context. This article addresses indications and attempts to analyze factors of importance in selecting patients for optimal long-term outcome, including the goals of comorbidity reduction and increase of quality-adjusted life years.

A critical difference between antiobesity surgery and other forms of surgery is that antiobesity surgery, in part, is "behavioral" surgery. It does

* Corresponding author.
E-mail address: jkral@downstate.edu (J.G. Kral).

0039-6109/05/$ - see front matter © 2005 Elsevier Inc. All rights reserved.
doi:10.1016/j.suc.2005.03.006

not have curative intent in the absence of any known etiology, and it is not reconstructive in the common meaning of the word. In addition, optimization of long-term "satisfactory outcome" requires significantly more pre- and postoperative patient education than most other surgery.

By its nature, antiobesity surgery alters the structure and function of the digestive tract, and affects its influence on intake and processing of food. The mechanisms behind the reduced food intake that are seen after antiobesity surgery are not entirely clear. One might argue that purely restrictive surgery, such as gastric banding (GB), simply reduces food intake by limiting intake; however, many patients report decreased appetite after the procedure. It also is not clear in which way antiobesity surgery so potently ameliorates the comorbidities that are associated with obesity, such as noninsulin-dependent diabetes mellitus (NIDDM) [2], asthma [3], and liver disease [4]. Emerging data suggest that altered gut peptide release after antiobesity surgery may influence food intake and cause amelioration of comorbidities. This is the topic of the second part of this article.

Indications

Before discussing indications for surgery, we need to analyze some of the basic premises for severely obese patients to seek antiobesity surgery (Box 1). Item 1 presupposes that an inability to control food intake is inherent in the condition of severe obesity. Binge-eating disorder (BED) is more prevalent and more severe with increasing body mass index (BMI) [5–7]. Item 2 includes exploring the patient's desire to reach a goal weight and ability to comprehend a realistic goal. It also is important to explore the patient's true motives and possible ambivalence about losing weight (Box 2). One also needs to assess possible psychosocial risk factors (Box 3). Of extra concern is the attitude, support, or potential codependency of a partner or spouse because weight loss seriously influences interpersonal relationships [8] as demonstrated in the authors' experience; break-up of partnerships is common postoperatively. There also is a need to make sure that the candidate fully comprehends the mechanisms behind the type of operation that is intended. If the procedure entails an obstructive component it is imperative that the

---

Box 1. Premises of candidacy for antiobesity surgery

1. Demonstrated inability to control food intake adequately.
2. Expression of real desire to lose weight.
3. Personal risk-benefit analysis comparing surgery to other treatment or non-treatment.
4. Personal cost-benefit analysis including cost of treatment of co-morbidity.

Box 2. Examples of motivational factors that influence candidacy for antiobesity surgery

Subjective benefits of being obese
Elicitation of help and pity (codependency)
Excuse for vocational/social failure or lack of competitiveness
Compensation for lack of competitiveness
Compensation for lack of assertiveness
Use of food for emotional comfort
Protection from unwanted sex
Avoidance of physical activity
Keeping warm in cold weather

---

candidate has learned and understood the rules of eating and vomiting (Box 4). The risk-benefit analysis in item 3 needs to be based on an understanding of the risks of remaining unoperated or treated by "medical" methods versus the benefits in net morbidity, prolongation of life, or improvement in quality of life (whether health-related or other) that are achieved after surgery. Trade-offs in quality of life before and after surgery need to be analyzed [9]. Item 4 includes the cost of nontreatment with its attendant present and future morbidity, which complicates the economic analysis.

Current and Future Indications for Surgery

Indications for surgery evolved during the 1980s and were formulated in the 1991 National Institutes of Health Consensus Development Conference, "Gastrointestinal Surgery for Severe Obesity" [10]. The recommendations largely emanated from increased awareness of the seriousness of obesity in terms of prevalence and morbidity, identification of the ineffectiveness of nonsurgical treatments, and improvements in safety of performance of antiobesity operations. In these new recommendations, the weight criterion for undergoing surgery, now expressed in terms of BMI, was broadened to include BMI of at least 35 kg/m^2 with manifest comorbidity. The requirement of a duration of obesity of 5 years or more was dropped in recognition of the fact that severe obesity takes many years to develop and often is of juvenile onset. Furthermore, the fact that candidates for antiobesity surgery have undergone a median of five to seven bouts of treatment before requesting surgical therapy resulted in the 1991 Consensus Statement suggesting that patients who seek treatment for the first time should be considered for nonsurgical treatment at the discretion of their physician [10].

The mandate to perform psychiatric evaluation was replaced by the proposal that a multidisciplinary team with surgical, medical, behavioral science, and nutritional expertise evaluate surgical candidates. Although

---

Box 3. Factors that influence postoperative complication rates and outcome in severely obese subjects

Positive
Employment
Married
Age younger than 40
Social support
Realistic expectations
Appointment-keeping
Diet compliance
Preoperative weight loss
Female sex
Quitting smoking
Knowledge of eating rules
Higher education

Negative
Minnesota multiphasic personality inventory psychopathology
Previous psychiatric admission
Negative life events
Alcohol, drug use
Black ethnicity
Codependent
Childhood abuse
Denial of disease
Secondary gain

---

there is no scientific evidence to support this seemingly reasonable approach to improve patient selection, the availability of such a multidisciplinary team postoperatively can benefit the long-term management of these patients. In the context of patient selection, the panel suggested that candidates for antiobesity surgery be evaluated with respect to their ability to comply adequately with the postoperative regimen; however, there is no scientifically validated method for performing such an evaluation.

The minimum recommended BMI criterion in the United States is 35 kg/m^2 in the presence of manifest serious comorbidity [10]. It is highly unlikely that any individual who has a body mass index of 30 or greater, sustained for more than 1 year, does not have evidence of comorbidity if evaluated thoroughly. Dyslipidemia, impaired glucose metabolism, fatty liver, and poor quality of life appear early in the natural history of obesity. In many European countries, patients who have a BMI of at least 35 kg/m^2 without demonstrated comorbidity are accepted for antiobesity surgery; the nationwide Swedish Obese Subjects (SOS) study, for example, accepts men

---

Box 4. Obligatory patient information before undergoing gastric operations for obesity

Rules of eating
Eat slowly with minimal stress and distraction
Progress your diet from liquids to semisolid food to solid food
Eat small portions
Chew well before swallowing
If you feel your pouch: stop eating
Don't drink with your food; drink between meals, waiting at least
  1 hour after eating

Rules of vomiting
If you vomit or regurgitate:
  Try to identify the reasons
  Don't drink for 4 hours
  Progress diet slowly
If nausea or vomiting during progression: nothing by mouth
  for 12 hours
If continuing vomiting, despite above measures: contact your
  doctor

---

with BMI of at least 34 kg/m^2 without requirement of diagnosed comorbidity [11]. With demonstration that the duration of exposure to obesity decreases the likelihood of sustainable remission or cure, an argument can be made for early intervention [12]. "Early", in this context, may be defined as shortly after attaining a critical BMI, in analogy with "early" treatment of diabetes [13]; however, it is not yet possible to define a critical BMI clearly for individual patients although lower BMI levels are increasingly being accepted [14,15] through recognition of the intractability of the disease, the need for prevention of comorbidity, and the significantly improved safety of the surgery following introduction of the laparoscopic approach [16]. Awareness of the serious impact of obesity on quality of life [17] and socioeconomic parameters [18] has helped to broaden the scope of factors that is included among indications for antiobesity surgery.

Setting age limits for surgery is complex. Few studies have examined the effect of childhood obesity on mortality. In one study of 508 lean or overweight adolescents (13 to 18 years old) who were followed for 55 years, overweight during adolescence was associated with an increased risk of mortality from all causes and an increased disease-specific mortality among men, but not women [19]. These data suggest a need for treatments that target childhood obesity.

Recent data demonstrate that a white male, age 20, with BMI of 40 kg/m^2 has approximately 6 years of life lost compared with a 60-year-old white male with the same BMI who has approximately 2 years of life lost. For white women, the differences in years of life lost due to differing BMI for the same age are not as clear. Thus, it can be argued that from a socioeconomic aspect, it is less favorable to operate on obese men who are older than 60 compared with younger men with the same BMI, whereas for women the data are less clear. In a recent study of mainly women, older patients (>60 years) demonstrated a higher pre- and postoperative comorbidity than younger patients. They also lost less weight; however, there was a significant improvement in comorbidities in the older patients [20]. Data in adolescents suggest that antiobesity surgery achieves favorable long-term outcome [21]. One can argue that the mandate to intervene early in young women, who may become pregnant, is even more compelling, owing to the risk of epigenetic transmission of obesity to offspring [22].

Classic predictors of treatment outcome, such as age, weight, and sex, have been studied with regard to antiobesity surgery. In a recent systematic review, 10 studies addressed age and outcome. The results were inconsistent; 6 studies found that younger patients lost more weight after surgery, whereas 4 did not. In terms of postoperative absolute weight loss, patients who were more overweight preoperatively lost less weight [23]. Male gender, older age, and high preoperative weight are risk factors for increased postoperative complications [24]. A simple office-based technique screened responders to a "nonmechanical" intervention, electrostimulation. Older age and lower BMI were among the positive predictors for weight loss [25].

Outcomes and patient selection

There are several different classes of outcomes after anti-obesity surgery; peri- and postoperative complications include side effects, comorbidity reduction, weight loss maintenance, economic changes, psychosocial changes and objective, and subjective quality of life changes. Many of these are interrelated and are associated with loss of body weight; however, weight loss alone is an inadequate outcome measure. Just as quality of life is multidimensional [17], so is the definition of successful outcome [26]; this makes it difficult to identify specific predictors that are useful for patient selection.

Five categories that are associated with poor long-term outcomes of antiobesity surgery have been identified: (1) poor patient knowledge; (2) psychosocial maladaptation; (3) anatomic complications; (4) gastrointestinal pathophysiology; and (5) weight-related symptomatology [27]. There is considerable interaction and overlap among these categories, but they are equally important to recognize and address in patient selection.

With regard to realistic expectations of maintained weight loss, there is considerable confusion about goal weights among surgeons [28] and other health-care professionals [29], which can influence the patient negatively. To confuse the picture further, several epidemiologic studies indicate that weight loss is associated with an increased risk of mortality [30]. This is paradoxical, because it is well-known that weight loss improves several risk factors for cardiovascular disease and NIDDM. In addition, reduced energy intake, which is a cornerstone in obesity treatment, extends life span in all investigated species [31].

Several explanations for the obesity–weight change–mortality paradox have been suggested. Many observational studies failed to record whether weight loss was intentional or unintentional [32,33]; however, recent data from the National Health Interview Survey found a lower mortality among subjects who intentionally lost weight. Conversely, unintentional weight loss was associated with a substantial increase in mortality [34]. It is important to be aware of this paradox because patients may have "been told by friends" that it is dangerous to lose weight. In addition, the minimum weight loss that is necessary to achieve optimal long-term outcome is not known. Data on overweight and obese subjects who have diabetes show that intentional weight loss reduces total mortality by 25%. An intentional weight reduction of 10 kg to 15 kg was associated with the largest mortality reduction (33%) [35]. Thus, a modest weight loss—from a mortality standpoint—might be sufficient, yet data from the SOS study demonstrate improved correction of diabetes and hypertension in patients who had greater weight loss from having undergone gastric bypass (GBP) compared with those who had vertical banded gastroplasty (VBG) [36]. With the commonly used operations today, it is reasonable to aim for an excess weight loss of 50% to 75% that is sustained for a minimum of 5 years.

An area of controversy that is relevant to evaluating obesity treatment is determining "appropriate," "sufficient," "healthy," or "optimal" weight goals for patients who are or have been severely obese. How much weight loss is "enough"? There is a widespread misconception that after surgery, a BMI of 30 kg/m^2 (still) represents an unhealthy body weight in patients who have lost weight and that the inability to bring patients under this arbitrary threshold constitutes "failure" of surgery. There is sufficient actuarial evidence, although sparse, to conclude that sustained voluntary weight loss is associated with decreased morbidity and mortality compared with that of the general population at the same level of BMI (or percent of "desirable" body weight"). Thus, it is not appropriate to conclude that patients with a BMI that is greater than 30 kg/m^2—whose BMI was at least 35 kg/m^2 or 40 kg/m^2 before surgery—are at similar risk of death or disease as those who never lost weight and exhibit "failure" of nonsurgical weight loss treatment.

Selective assignment

Most surgeons who are engaged in antiobesity surgery have adopted one particular operation that they tend to use exclusively, with no regard for individualization. Many of the failures are not solely technical, but are based on poor patient selection and the inability to identify outcome predictors. Previous discussion has focused on selecting surgical candidates, but is it possible to match a particular patient with a specific surgical procedure?

In the search for predictors of outcome after antiobesity surgery, the effect of preoperative eating behavior has been studied. In one study, "sweet eaters" fared less well after gastric restrictive surgery compared with "nonsweet eaters" [37]; however, several studies demonstrated that sweet eaters and nonsweet eaters are equally successful in terms of weight loss after gastric restrictive procedures [38–40]. It is indisputable, however, that maladaptive eating (such as the "soft calorie syndrome") adversely affects the outcomes of purely restrictive operations.

Eating behavior, assessed by the three factor eating questionnaire (TFEQ), has been used as a predictor of postoperative weight loss. Patients who ate in response to "pleasant feelings" lost more weight than those who ate in response to "stress" [41]. Furthermore, there was a negative correlation between "disinhibition" in the TEFQ and percentage of weight lost [42]. Thus, although some eating behavior data may predict post-operative outcome, it seems difficult to allocate patients to different surgical procedures based on preoperative eating behavior; however, many surgeons allocate patients with high consumption of liquid carbohydrates to bypass surgery in the belief that these patients might be deterred from consuming liquid carbohydrates because of dumping-like symptoms, reported by some patients. Cultural differences in eating behavior, such as those between Europe, Australia, and the United States, also may account for differences in outcome. Purely gastric restrictive procedures tend to do better in Europe and Australia than in the United States [43–45] and biliopancreatic diversion (BPD) does better in Italy than in the United States [46]. One might speculate that this is due to differences in preoperative BMI (Europeans tend to be less heavy), dietary intake (pasta versus fast food), snacking, and formal family dining.

Regarding BED, there are some data to guide patient allocation to different surgical procedures. Two retrospective studies suggested that BED is a negative predictor [47,48], whereas three prospective studies have not been able to demonstrate a correlation between BED and postoperative outcome [38,49,50]. One retrospective study suggested that BPD might correct BED [51]. These types of reports have not taken into consideration the fact that all gastric operations, at least during the first postoperative year, create such restriction that it is physically impossible for patients to fulfill criteria for binge eating. Although the BED might be "improved" temporarily, it is difficult to conclude that the condition which underlies the disorder is "cured"!

Recently, mutations in the melanocortin receptor–4 (MCR4) gene have been implicated in BED [52]. Although these results are controversial with respect to functionality of the polymorphisms in vitro [53,54], subsequent findings imply the existence of loss-of-function in other relevant pathways. Regardless of this "controversy," outcomes 3 years after GB in 300 patients clearly demonstrated poorer weight loss, less amelioration of comorbidity, and more complications in patients who had MC4R mutations and in patients who had BED and no mutations [55]. A small subset of patients that had polymorphisms and was converted to GBP seem to have poorer weight loss than those without. It is too early to determine an optimal strategy for patients who have BED with or without gene abnormalities. Nevertheless, surgical treatment is still more effective than any other method in this context; there is no reason to conclude that BED is a contraindication for antiobesity surgery.

Patients who have gastroesophageal reflux disease are treated best by bypass surgery, although several studies documented improvement after restrictive procedures [56,57]; however, most studies found no change postoperatively or aggravation of the disease after gastric restrictive procedures [58,59]. These differences likely are due to variations in pouch size that result in varying amounts of secretory mucosa above the restriction.

Physiology of gastrointestinal antiobesity operations

The goal of antiobesity surgery is to enhance satiety or reduce hunger signals to create undernutrition [60]. Purely gastric restrictive procedures (ie, limiting food intake by way of reservoir capacity and rate of emptying), such as VBG and GB, cause gastric or esophageal distention which elicits early satiety, nausea, discomfort, or even vomiting when pouch capacity has been exceeded. The esophagus is well-characterized in regards to neuropeptide distribution [61]. Recent positron emission tomography studies of esophageal afferents have identified brain loci that are stimulated by distention [62]. These loci are in proximity to loci that are stimulated by appetitive behavior [63]. Hypothetically, esophageal signals could participate in regulating (inhibiting) food intake. Gastric distention of the cardia/upper stomach also demonstrated increased activity in areas that are involved in appetite regulation [64]. In line with this finding, a recent article demonstrates that optimal restriction—in weight stable subjects after GB—evokes greater satiety than does reduced restriction [65]. There are few studies of meal-stimulated plasma concentrations of gut hormones after gastric restrictive surgery [66]. Recent data demonstrate that plasma ghrelin [67] and peptide YY (PYY) [68] increase after gastric restrictive surgery, whereas leptin decreases [65]. These changes most likely are secondary to reduced body weight because these hormones are known to fluctuate with body weight. It is unclear whether this has any impact on appetite.

To examine the role of afferent and efferent vagal signals and their contribution to weight loss, truncal vagotomy alone (ie, without drainage) was studied in a small group of obese patients [69]. Because of the modest short-term weight loss in comparison with other procedures, vagotomy was abandoned as a single procedure; however, based on findings of amelioration of calorically dense liquid intake [70]—the hallmark of the "soft calorie syndrome" and the primary cause of failure of gastric restrictive procedures [71]—vagotomy was combined with gastroplasty in another set of patients. Vagotomy potentiated the weight loss after VBG [72]. The vagus ("wide-ranging") nerve has numerous functions that affect appetitive behavior. Although efferent or motor effects only involve 20% of vagal fibers, these effects are best studied and most familiar to surgeons. Vagal afferents relay important sensory information of particular interest in the context of energy balance and ingestive behavior. Thus, abdominal truncal vagotomy has wide-ranging effects on thirst and hunger that are relevant for antiobesity surgery.

Discovery of the only peripheral orexigenic peptide (ghrelin) [73] has stimulated interest in mechanisms that underlie the weight-reducing effects of GBP. Initially, the operation relies on gastric restriction much like gastroplasty (6–18 months). Subsequently, when the pouch and stoma have stretched, other mechanisms take effect to maintain the loss and account for the superior weight loss maintenance as compared with purely restrictive operations. The appetitive mechanisms of the diversionary component of GBP are achieved through the absence of a pyloric "meter" or "brake" and allow rapid transit by way of the gastrojejunostomy, and maldigestion that is caused by the absence of acid and pepsin and the grinding-mixing forces of the stomach. Thus, undigested food that is shunted rapidly into the small bowel can cause nimiety by way of mechanoreceptors, and possibly, satiety by way of chemoreceptors [74] or neurohumoral mechanisms.

GBP causes profound changes in plasma gut peptide levels from the altered anatomy. Ghrelin, secreted mainly from the stomach, has been suggested to be a meal stimulatory peptide [75]. It is decreased after GBP surgery in some studies [76a], unchanged in some studies (despite weight loss) [76], but increased in other studies [77]. There has been a renewed interest in PYY after administration of truncated PYY3-36 was shown to decrease food intake in obese humans [78]. PYY levels increase post-prandially after GBP surgery [79]. Glucagon-like peptide–1 (GLP-1) is secreted, like PYY, by the L cells of the distal gut in response to a meal. GLP-1 also decreases food intake and appetite in obese subjects [80]. GLP-1 has not been measured specifically after food intake after GBP, but because plasma concentrations of enteroglucagon are elevated after GBP [66], and enteroglucagon and GLP-1 are secreted in parallel from the L-cells of the gut, it is reasonable to assume that plasma concentrations of GLP-1 also might be elevated, and thus, decrease appetite. One study found that fasting GLP-1 concentrations were not elevated 3 weeks after GBP [81].

Compared with gastric restriction, the improved weight loss after GBP may be attributed to increased secretion of satiating peptides or impaired secretion of the orexigenic peptide, ghrelin, from bypass of the foregut through unknown mechanisms. Infusion of nutrients into the stomach, duodenum, or jejunum resulted in the same degree of ghrelin suppression [82]. In addition, a small degree of malabsorption with early delivery of nutrients to the hindgut increases the release of GLP-1 and PYY, which, in turn, may induce a prolonged and increased satiety response [83]. The profound effect of GBP on NIDDM [12] also may be attributed to changes in plasma concentrations of GLP-1 and ghrelin [83]. As an incretin, GLP-1 is insulinotropic and inhibits the release of glucagon, and thus, decreases plasma glucose concentrations [80,84].

Gastrointestinal polypeptide patterns have been studied after intestinal bypass operations with varying lengths of jejunum and ileum in continuity [85–87]. Although these operations no longer are performed as primary procedures for surgical treatment of obesity, their effects on gut peptides are relevant and the information provided can be used in developing other strategies for weight control. GLP-1 and PYY concentrations are elevated short-term (9 months) and long-term (20 years) after jejunoileal bypass (JIB), and likely contribute to satiety after JIB [88,89]. Further support for the importance of these peptides in contributing to the weight loss that is seen after antiobesity surgery is the fact that ileal interposition results in increased plasma concentrations of PYY and GLP-1, which is accompanied by weight loss in the rat [90,91] and dogs [92].

The most extensive gastrointestinal operation for obesity is BPD [93] and its pylorus-sparing modification, duodenal switch (BPD-DS) [94–96]. Analyses of peptide patterns after BPD were performed in the early 1980s and demonstrated increased plasma enteroglucagon levels [85]. More recent studies by the same group showed that ghrelin levels increase after BPD [97]. Enteroglucagon levels in patients after duodenal switch were increased and give an indirect indication of mechanisms that explain weight loss after BPD-DS [98].

One often forgotten aspect of appetite control and obesity surgery is the role of fatty acid secretion from lipolysis and ketone body production from catabolism during rapid weight loss. Free fatty acids and ketone bodies inhibit food intake in mammals [99]. In addition, "starvation" itself is a stressor that results in increased plasma cortisol levels, and release of cytokines from adipose tissue, both of which may have centrally mediated appetite-reducing effects. During fasting, cortisol is related inversely to ghrelin [100] and cortisone induces leptin gene expression which results in reduced food intake in rodents [101].

Summary

Antiobesity surgery works through simple principles that affect ingestion (restriction), assimilation and storage (bypass), and desire to ingest (satiation and aversion) nutrients. Ideally, the goal is to achieve "programmed" or controlled undernutrition [60]. It fails through maladaptive eating behavior more often than technical inadequacy. Rather than speculating over mechanisms for optimizing physiologic responses which influence weight regulation, increased efforts should be directed toward preoperative assessment and treatment of existing impediments to normalization of eating behavior and toward identification of risk factors for the development of maladaptive eating postoperatively. Antiobesity surgery can contribute to the understanding of neurohumoral signals that are involved in appetite regulation by creating models to test the relative importance of different segments of the gastrointestinal tract (upper versus lower gut signals). Antiobesity surgery also can shed light on the pathophysiology of obesity through studies before, during, and after restoration of physiologically appropriate levels of body weight.

References

[1] American College of Surgeons. ACS statement on principles underlying perioperative responsibility. Bull Am Coll Surg 1996;81:39.

[2] Buchwald H, Avidor Y, Braunwald E, et al. Bariatric surgery: a systematic review and meta-analysis. JAMA 2004;292:1724–37.

[3] Dixon JB, Chapman L, O'Brien PE. Marked improvement in asthma after Lap-Band surgery for morbid obesity. Obes Surg 1999;9:385–9.

[4] Kral JG, Thung SN, Biron S, et al. Effects of surgical treatment of the metabolic syndrome of liver fibrosis and cirrhosis. Surgery 2004;135:48–58.

[5] Telch CF, Agras WS, Rossiter EM. Binge eating with increasing adiposity. Int J Eat Disord 1988;7:115–9.

[6] Kral JG. Morbidity of severe obesity. Surg Clin North Am 2001;81:1039–61.

[7] Guss JL, Kissileff HR, Devlin MJ, et al. Binge size increases with body mass index in women with binge-eating disorder. Obes Res 2002;10:1021–9.

[8] Hafner RJ, Rogers J. Husbands' adjustment to wives' weight loss after gastric restriction for morbid obesity. Int J Obes 1990;14:1069–78.

[9] Rand CSW, Macgregor AMC. Successful weight loss following surgery and the perceived liability of morbid obesity. Int J Obes 1991;15:577–9.

[10] National Institutes of Health Consensus Development Panel. Gastrointestinal surgery for severe obesity. Ann Int Med 1991;115:956–61.

[11] Sjöström L, Larsson B, Backman L, et al. Swedish Obese Subjects (SOS). Recruitment for an intervention study and selected description of the obese state. Int J Obes 1992;16:465–79.

[12] Pories WJ, Swanson MS, MacDonald KG, et al. Who would have thought it? An operation proves to be the most effective therapy for adult onset diabetes mellitus. Ann Surg 1995;222:339–50.

[13] Banerji MA, Chaiken RL, Lebovitz HE. Prolongation of near normoglycemic remission in black NIDDM subjects with chronic low-dose sulfonylurea treatment. Diabetes 1995;44:466–70.

[14] Angrisani L, Favretti F, Furbetta F, et al. Italian group for Lap-Band system: results of a multicenter study on patients with BMI < or = 35 kg/m². Obes Surg 2004;14:415–8.

[15] O'Brien P, Dixon J, Laurie C, et al. A randomized controlled trial of medical versus surgical therapy in the management of obesity. Obes Res 2004;12(Suppl):A33.

[16] Nguyen NT, Goldman C, Rosenquist CJ, et al. Laparoscopic versus open gastric bypass: a randomized study of outcomes, quality of life and costs. Ann Surg 2001;234:279–89.

[17] Kral JG, Sjöström LV, Sullivan MBE. Assessment of quality of life before and after surgery for surgical obesity. Am J Clin Nutr 1992;55:611s–4s.

[18] Narbro K, Ågren G, Jonsson E, et al. Sick leave and disability pension before and after treatment for obesity: a report from the Swedish Obese Subjects (SOS) study. Int J Obes 1999;23:619–24.

[19] Must A, Jacques PF, Dallal GE, et al. Long-term morbidity and mortality of overweight adolescents. A follow-up of the Harvard Growth Study of 1922–1935. N Engl J Med 1992; 327:1350–5.

[20] Sugerman HJ, DeMaria EJ, Kellum JM, et al. Effects of bariatric surgery in older patients. Ann Surg 2004;240:243–7.

[21] Rand CSW, Macgregor AMC. Adolescents having obesity surgery: a 6-year follow-up. South Med J 1994;87:1208–13.

[22] Kral JG. Preventing and treating obesity in girls and young women to curb the epidemic. Obes Res 2004;12:1539–46.

[23] Herpertz S, Kielmann R, Wolf AM, et al. Do psychosocial variables predict weight loss or mental health after obesity surgery? A systematic review. Obes Res 2004;12: 1554–69.

[24] Livingston EH, Huerta S, Arthur D, et al. Male gender is a predictor of morbidity and age a predictor of mortality for patients undergoing gastric bypass surgery. Ann Surg 2002;236: 576–82.

[25] Shikora SA. The U.S. experience with implantable gastric stimulation (IGS) for the treatment of obesity–update on the ongoing clinical trials. Obes Surg 2004;14(Suppl 1): S40–8.

[26] Brolin RE. Critical analysis of results: weight loss and quality of data. Am J Clin Nutr 1992; 55:577s–81s.

[27] Knol JA. Management of the problem patient after bariatric surgery. Gastroenterol Clin N Am 1994;23:345–69.

[28] MacLean LD, Rhode BM, Nohr CW. Late outcome of isolated gastric bypass. Ann Surg 2000;231:524–8.

[29] Hsu LKG, Benotti PN, Dwyer J, et al. Nonsurgical factors that influence the outcome of bariatric surgery. a review. Psychosom Med 1998;60:338–46.

[30] Khaodhiar L, Blackburn GL. Health benefits and risks of weight loss. In: Björntorp P, editor. International textbook of obesity. Chichester (UK): John Wiley & Sons, Ltd; 2001. p. 413–39.

[31] Walford RL, Harris SB, Weindruch R. Dietary restriction and aging: historical phases, mechanisms and current directions. J Nutr 1987;117:1650–4.

[32] Meltzer AA, Everhart JE. Unintentional weight loss in the United States. Am J Epidemiol 1995;142:1039–46.

[33] Williamson DF. Intentional weight loss: patterns in the general population and its association with morbidity and mortality. Int J Obes 1997;21(Suppl 1):S14–9.

[34] Gregg EW, Gerzoff RB, Thompson TJ, et al. Intentional weight loss and death in overweight and obese US adults 35 years of age and older. Ann Intern Med 2003;138:383–9.

[35] Williamson DF, Thompson TJ, Thun M, et al. Intentional weight loss and mortality among overweight individuals with diabetes. Diabetes Care 2000;23:1499–504.

[36] Sjöström CD, Peltonen M, Wedel H, et al. Differentiated long-term effects of intentional weight loss on diabetes and hypertension. Hypertension 2000;36:20–5.

[37] Sugerman HJ, Londrey GL, Kellum JM, et al. Weight loss with vertical banded gastroplasty and Roux-Y gastric bypass for morbid obesity with selective versus random assignment. Am J Surg 1989;157:93–102.

[38] Busetto L, Valente P, Pisent C, et al. Eating pattern in the first year following adjustable silicone gastric banding (ASGB) for morbid obesity. Int J Obes 1996;20:539–46.

[39] Lindroos AK, Lissner L, Sjöström L. Weight change in relation to intake of sugar and sweet foods before and after weight reducing gastric surgery. Int J Obes 1996;20:634–43.

[40] Hudson SM, Dixon JB, O'Brien PE. Sweet eating is not a predictor after Lap-Band placement: can we finally bury the myth? Obes Res 2002;12:789–94.

[41] Gentry K, Halverson JD, Heisler S. Psychologic assessment of morbidly obese patients undergoing gastric bypass: a comparison of preoperative and post-operative adjustment. Surgery 1984;95:215–20.

[42] Delin CR, Watts JM, Bassett DL. An exploration of the outcomes of gastric bypass surgery for morbid obesity: patient characteristics and indices of success. Obes Res 1995;5:159–70.

[43] Näslund E, Backman L, Granström L, et al. Seven year results of vertical banded gastroplasty for morbid obesity. Eur J Surg 1997;163:281–6.

[44] Cordera F, Mail JL, Thompson GB, et al. Unsatisfactory weight loss after vertical banded gastroplasty: is conversion to Roux-en-Y gastric bypass successful? Surgery 2004;136:731–7.

[45] O'Brien PE, Dixon JB. Laparoscopic adjustable gastric banding in the treatment of morbid obesity. Arch Surg 2003;138:376–82.

[46] Scopinaro N, Adami GF, Marinari GM, et al. Biliopancreatic diversion. World J Surg 1998;22:936–46.

[47] Pekkarinen T, Koskela K, Huikuri K, et al. Long-term results of gastroplasty for morbid obesity: binge-eating as a predictor of outcome. Obes Res 1994;4:248–55.

[48] Mitchell JE, Lancaster KL, Burgard MA, et al. Long-term follow-up of patients' status after gastric bypass. Obes Surg 2001;11:464–8.

[49] Busetto L, Segato G, De Marchi F, et al. Outcome predictors in morbidly obese recipients of an adjustable gastric band. Obes Surg 2002;12:83–92.

[50] Powers PS, Perez A, Boyd F, et al. Eating pathology before and after bariatric surgery: a prospective study. Int J Eat Disord 1999;25:293–300.

[51] Adami GF, Gandolfo P, Scopinaro N. Binge eating in obesity. Int J Obes 1996;20:793–4.

[52] Branson R, Potoczna N, Kral JG, et al. Binge eating as a major phenotype of melanocortin 4 receptor gene mutation. N Engl J Med 2003;343:1096–103.

[53] Herpertz S, Siffert W, Hebebrand J. Lack of association of melanocortin-4 gene mutations and binge eating disorder. N Engl J Med 2003;349:6.

[54] Farooqi IS, Keogh JM, Yeo GS, et al. Clinical spectrum of obesity and mutations in the melanocortin 4 receptor gene. N Engl J Med 2003;348:1085–95.

[55] Potoczna N, Branson R, Kral JG, et al. Gene variants and binge eating as predictors of comorbidity and outcome of treatment in severe obesity. J Gastrointest Surg 2004;8:971–82.

[56] Dixon JB, O'Brien PE. Gastroesophageal reflux in obesity: the effect of lap-band placement. Obes Surg 1999;9:527–31.

[57] Deitel M, Khanna R, Hagen J, et al. Vertical banded gastroplasty as an antireflux procedure. Am J Surg 1988;155:512–6.

[58] Näslund E, Granström L, Melcher A, et al. Gastroesophageal reflux before and after vertical banded gastroplasty in the treatment of obesity. Eur J Surg 1996;162:303–6.

[59] Ortega J, Escudero MD, Mora F, et al. Outcome of esophageal function and 24-hour esophageal pH monitoring after vertical banded gastroplasty and Roux-en-Y gastric bypass. Obes Surg 2004;14:1086–94.

[60] Cannizzo F, Kral JG. Obesity surgery: a model of programmed undernutrition. Curr Opin Clin Nutr Metab Care 1998;1:363–8.

[61] Wattachow DA, Furness JB, Costa M, et al. Distribution of neuropeptides in the human esophagus. Gastroentrology 1987;93:1363–71.

[62] Aziz Q, Andersson JL, Valind S, et al. Identification of human brain loci processing esophageal sensation using positron emission tomography. Gastroenterology 1997;113:50–9.

[63] Tataranni PA, Gautier JF, Chen K, et al. Neuroanatomical correlates of hunger and satiation in humans using positron emission tomography. Proc Natl Acad Sci USA 1999;96:4569–74.

[64] Stephan E, Parado JV, Faris PL, et al. Functional neuroimaging of gastric distention. J Gastrointest Surg 2003;7:740–9.

[65] Dixon AF, Dixon JB, O'Brien PE. Laparoscopic adjustable gastric banding induces prolonged satiety: a randomised blind crossover study. J Clin Endocrinol Metab 2005; 90(2):813–9.

[66] Kellum JM, Kuemmerle JF, O'Dorisio TM, et al. Gastrointestinal hormone responses to meals before and after gastric bypass and vertical banded gastroplasty. Ann Surg 1990;211:763–70.

[67] Nijhuis J, van Dielen FM, Buurman WA, et al. Ghrelin, leptin and insulin levels after restrictive surgery: a 2-year follow-up study. Obes Surg 2004;14:783–7.

[68] Alvarez Bartolome M, Borque M, Martinez-Sarmiento J, et al. Peptide YY secretion in morbidly obese patients before and after vertical banded gastroplasty. Obes Surg 2002;12: 324–7.

[69] Kral JG. Vagotomy as a treatment for severe obesity. Lancet 1978;I:307–8.

[70] Görtz L, Björkman A-C, Andersson H, et al. Truncal vagotomy reduces food and liquid intake in man. Physiol Behav 1990;48:779–81.

[71] Kral JG, Kissileff HR. Surgical approaches to the treatment of obesity. Ann Behav Med 1987;9:15–9.

[72] Kral JG, Görtz L, Hermanson G, et al. Gastroplasty for obesity: long-term weight loss improved by vagotomy. World J Surg 1993;17:75–9.

[73] Asakawa A, Inui A, Kaga T, et al. Ghrelin is an appetite-stimulatory signal from stomach with structural resemblance to motilin. Gastroenterology 2001;120:337–45.

[74] Mei N. Intestinal chemosensitivity. Physiol Rev 1985;65:211–37.

[75] Cummings DE, Purnell JQ, Frayo RS, et al. A preprandial rise in plasma ghrelin levels suggests a role in meal initiation in humans. Diabetes 2001;50:1714–9.

[76] Faraj M, Havel PJ, Phelis S, et al. Plasma acylation-stimulating protein, adiponectin, leptin, and ghrelin before and after weight loss induced by gastric bypass surgery in morbidly obese subjects. J Clin Endocrinol Metab 2003;88:1594–602.

[76a] Cummings DE, Weigle DS, Fray RS, et al. Plasma ghrelin levels after diet-induced weight loss or gastric bypass surgery. N Engl J Med 2002;346:1623–30.

[77] Holdstock C, Engström BE, Öhrvall M, et al. Ghrelin and adipose regulatory peptides: effect of gastric bypass surgery in obese humans. J Clin Endocrinol Metab 2003;88:3177–83.

[78] Batterham RL, Cohen MA, Ellis SM, et al. Inhibition of food intake in obese subjects by peptide YY3–36. N Engl J Med 2003;349:941–8.

[79] Korner J, Bessler M, Cirilo L, et al. Effects of Roux-en-Y gastric bypass surgery on fasting and postprandial concentrations of plasma ghrelin, PYY and insulin. J Clin Endocrinol Metab 2005;90(1):359–65.

[80] Näslund E, Barkeling B, King N, et al. Energy intake and appetite are suppressed by glucagon-like peptide-1 (GLP-1) in obese men. Int J Obes 1999;23:304–11.

[81] Rubino F, Gagner M, Gentileschi P, et al. The early effect of the Roux-en-Y gastric bypass on hormones involved in body weight regulation and glucose metabolism. Ann Surg 2004; 240:236–42.

[82] Overduin J, Frayo RS, Grill HJ, et al. Role of duodenum and macronutrient type in ghrelin regulation. Endocrinology 2004; Epub ahead of print.

[83] Cummings DE, Overduin J, Foster-Schubert KE. Gastric bypass for obesity: mechanisms of weight loss and diabetes resolution. J Clin Endocrinol Metab 2004;89:2608–15.

[84] Holst JJ. Glucagon-like peptide-1: a newly discovered gastrointestinal hormone. Gastroenterology 1994;107:1848–55.

[85] Sarson DL, Scopinaro N, Bloom SR. Gut hormone changes after jejunoileal bypass (JIB) or biliopancreatic (BPB) bypass surgery for morbid obesity. Int J Obes 1981;5:471–80.

[86] Sørensen TI, Lauritsen KB, Holst JJ, et al. Gut and pancreatic hormones after jejunoileal bypass with 3:1 or 1:3 jejunoileal ratio. Digestion 1983;26:137–45.

[87] Kral JG. Malabsorptive procedures in surgical treatment of morbid obesity. Gastroenterol Clin North Am 1987;16:293–305.

[88] Näslund E, Grybäck P, Backman L, et al. Distal small bowel gut hormones: correlation to fasting antroduodenal motility and gastric emptying. Dig Dis Sci 1998;43:945–53.

[89] Näslund E, Grybäck P, Hellström PM, et al. Gastrointestinal hormones and gastric emptying 20 years after jejunoileal bypass for massive obesity. Int J Obes 1997;48:387–92.

[90] Strader AD, Vahl TP, Jandacek RJ, et al. Weight loss through ileal transposition is accompanied by increased ileal hormone secretion and synthesis in the rat. Am J Physiol Endocrinol Metab 2005;288(2):E447–53.

[91] Koopmans HS, Ferri GL, Sarson DL, et al. The effects of ileal transposition and jejunoileal bypass on food intake and GI hormone levels in rats. Physiol Behav 1984;33:601–9.

[92] Smithy WB, Caudros CL, Johnson H, et al. Effects of ileal transposition on body weight and intestinal morphology in dogs. Int J Obes 1986;10:453–60.

[93] Scopinaro N, Gianetta E, Adami GF, et al. Biliopancreatic diversion for obesity at eighteen years. Surgery 1996;119:261–8.

[94] Welch NT, Yasui A, Kim CB, et al. Effect of duodenal switch procedure on gastric acid production, intragastric pH, gastric emptying, and gastrointestinal hormones. Am J Surg 1992;163:37–44.

[95] Hess DS, Hess DW. Biliopancreatic diversion with duodenal switch. Obes Surg 1998;8:267–82.

[96] Marceau P, Hould FS, Simard S, et al. Biliopancreatic diversion with duodenal switch. World J Surg 1998;22:947–54.

[97] Adami GF, Cordera R, Andragehetti G, et al. Changes in serum ghrelin concentrations following biliopancreatic diversion for obesity. Obes Res 2004;12:684–7.

[98] Wilson P, Welch NT, Hinder RA, et al. Abnormal plasma gut hormones in pathologic duodenogastric reflux and their response to surgery. Am J Surg 1993;165:169–76.

[99] Scharrer E. Control of food intake by fatty acid oxidation and ketogenesis. Nutrition 1999;15:704–14.

[100] Espelund U, Hansen TK, Højlund K, et al. Fasting unmasks a strong inverse association between ghrelin and cortisol in serum: studies in obese and normal-weight subjects. J Clin Endocrinol Metab 2005;90(2):741–6.

[101] De Vos P, Saladin R, Auwerx J, et al. Induction of ob gene expression by corticosteroids is accompanied by weight loss and reduced food intake. J Biol Chem 1995;270:15958–61.

SURGICAL
CLINICS OF
NORTH AMERICA

Surg Clin N Am 85 (2005) 741–755

Psychologic Issues in Bariatric Surgery—the Surgeon's Perspective

Nancy Puzziferri, MD[a,b,*]

[a]Assistant Professor of Surgery, University of Texas Southwestern School of Medicine,
5323 Harry Hines Boulevard, Dallas, TX 75390, USA
[b]Staff Surgeon, VA North Texas Health Care System, 4500 S. Lancaster Road,
Dallas, TX 75216, USA

Why do psychologic issues matter?

The consensus that obesity surgery is superior to medical intervention is growing and is supported by abundant evidence. Most patients lose a significant amount of weight, maintain their weight loss long-term, and therefore have improved quality of life with decreased comorbidities and enhanced psychosocial functioning. Despite these benefits from surgery, 5% to 30% of patients lose little weight or are unable to maintain their weight loss postoperatively. Although bariatric surgery is now relatively safe, it is elective, and any risks incurred should not be undertaken unless the chance for success has been optimized and is favorable.

Gastric bypass and banding have been referred to as tools to be used by obese patients. The success of these procedures, outside of medical complications, relies on patients' following prescribed diets. Any patient can override the constraints of a gastric pouch and block weight loss by sipping on high-caloric-density liquids throughout the day. The contribution of behavior to the success of weight loss surgery cannot be overlooked. Unfortunately, it is this component that has been so difficult to define in terms of affecting or predicting outcome.

Lacking are validated predictors for success and standardized preoperative psychologic assessment tools.

Surgeons are not often in a situation that warrants or supports long-term follow-up of patients. Long-term follow-up is essential when, at 18 months after surgery, a significant portion of bariatric patients begin to regain

* Correspondence. University of Texas Southwestern School of Medicine, 5323 Harry Hines Boulevard, Dallas, TX 75390.
E-mail address: Nancy.Puzziferri@utsouthwestern.edu

0039-6109/05/$ - see front matter © 2005 Elsevier Inc. All rights reserved.
doi:10.1016/j.suc.2005.04.003
surgical.theclinics.com

weight. Follow-up also is needed for those who are not losing the expected weight in the first year after surgery. The evolving needs of the formerly obese patient can be addressed optimally in the context of a multidisciplinary team of mental health care professionals, nutritionists, exercise physiologists, and nurses.

Psychologic characteristics of obese patients

Overview

Obese patients have been well characterized psychologically. Although in the United States they carry a psychologic burden in the suffering generated from prejudice and discrimination [1], they do not have an increased prevalence of psychopathology compared with normal-weight patients [2–4]. This is not to say that the obese do not have psychologic disturbances specific to them but rather that standardized tests may not detect problems such as disturbed body image or diet induced stress [5]. Obese individuals do exhibit psychologic ailments that are consistent with those seen in persons subjected to prejudice and discrimination [6–9].

The obese population, like the general population, is heterogeneous. The subset of obese patients who seek and ultimately undergo surgical treatment have, in some studies, been shown to possess more psychologic pathology than their counterparts [10,11]. It is thought that although the obese as a group do not have more psychopathology than normal-weight individuals, those selected for surgery do [12]. Despite identifiable psychopathology in 58% of patients at preoperative evaluation, at least 80% are approved for surgery. Reasons for rejection are overt untreated psychiatric illness, severe situational stress, active substance abuse, insufficient motivation or understanding to comply with postoperative guidelines, demonstrated noncompliance with previous medical care, or lack of adequate environmental support [13,14].

Psychiatric disorders

Axis I disorders are readily discernable by a number of survey and behavioral assessments. Black and colleagues [15] studied 88 obese patients for prevalence of psychiatric disorders. They found lifetime prevalence rates of 20% for major depression, 23% for alcohol abuse or dependency, 41% for psychosexual dysfunction, and 48% for tobacco dependency. Simple phobia, general anxiety, and posttraumatic stress disorder each occurred in 16% of the cohort. The prevalence of any axis II disorders was 56%: 49% cluster A (eccentric), 29% cluster B (dramatic, excluding narcissistic), and 5% cluster C (anxious, including avoidant and passive-aggressive).

Fifteen studies reviewed for prevalence and type of mental illness in the obese showed rates of 4% to 80% for depression and 15% to 83% for personality disorders [15]. These prevalences may be no different than in the general population. Morbid obesity is a risk factor for development of a mood disorder [16], and obese women are more susceptible than obese men to mood disorders [17].

Eating disorders

Binge eating disorder is defined as consumption of an objectively large quantity of food in a brief period (<2 hours) during which the patient experiences a subjective loss of control and significant emotional stress. This consumption is not followed by vomiting; binge eating plus vomiting constitute bulimia nervosa. This behavior must occur on average at least 2 days/wk for at least 6 months. The prevalence of binge eating disorder in obese patients is 20% to 30%, versus 2% in normal-weight patients [18]. Thirty percent to 68% of obese patients report binge eating problems but do not meet full criteria for binge eating disorder. Binge eating is responsive to cognitive and behavioral treatment as well as to medication.

The prevalence of bulimia nervosa in the obese is similar to that in the general population [19]. Bulimia nervosa is characterized by binge eating followed by self-induced vomiting, fasting, exercise, or excessive use of laxatives, enemas, or diuretics. Because vomiting after gastric bypass surgery may differ in significance from vomiting induced preoperatively, the symptom must be interpreted in context. Vomiting is the most frequent complication after restrictive procedures. Barring surgical complication, vomiting is usually caused by eating a food volume in excess of pouch size or by eating inappropriate foods. Vomiting that persists because the patient knowingly engages in inappropriate eating behavior may represent a failed attempt at binging [20].

Although an obese patient may not meet strict criteria for the diagnosis of an eating disorder, similar characteristics do exist. These similarities include dissatisfaction with the body or negative body view, frequent dieting, and experiences of failure related to eating and eating restraint (eating according to weight goals versus physiologic cues) [21].

Eating patterns

Eating rates and patterns of obese persons differ from those of lean patients. Women with central obesity and obese males eat at a faster rate than controls [22]. Obese patients can eat greater volumes of all types of foods and eat until all food served is gone. Normal-weight patients stop eating when they feel full, regardless of the amount of food served [23]. Everyday patterns of eating associated with weight gain include eating rapidly, eating when not hungry, and consuming large amounts of high-calorie beverages [24].

Restrained eaters eat according to cognitive aspirations, that is, at frequencies and in amounts consistent with their weight goals. The emphasis is turned away from perceiving physiologic or psychologic pressures to eat. This eating pattern is the one seen in weight-loss diets. Restrained eaters are found among normal-weight individuals and the obese but, because they diet more often, are thought to exist in greater numbers in those who are overweight. It is not known if preoccupation with weight leads to restrained eating or if restrained eating leads to preoccupation of weight. Once guiding cognitive aspirations are lifted, restrained eaters eat more than unrestrained eaters [25].

Night-eating syndrome refers to an eating pattern seen in 8% to 33% of obese patients. The key features are excessive eating at night, morning anorexia, and general insomnia, but morning anorexia may be absent [26–28]. Additionally, a phenomenon called "sleep eating" occurs in 9% to 27% of the obese population [29]. Sleep eating consists of rising after the onset of sleep to eat large amounts of high-calorie foods.

Many obese patients are frequently engaged in a weight-loss diet. These continued and ineffective efforts at dieting contribute to a sense of failure. Depression with weight-loss dieting is a recognized phenomenon [12,26,30].

Prejudice and discrimination

Prejudice toward overweight individuals is the last socially acceptable form of prejudice [31]. The perception is that obese individuals cause their obesity. Weight can and should be controlled. When it is not, the overweight person is thought to be to blame. Stigmatization begins as early as age 6 years, when overweight children are seen as lazy, dirty, stupid, ugly, cheats, and liars [1]. Nearly all patients report being teased or receiving negative comments. Eighty percent of the obese report mistreatment related to their weight [7]. Health care professionals are included among those who misunderstand, ridicule, and reject the obese. Such treatment contributes to low self-esteem and self-appraisal, poor interpersonal relationships, and depressive reactions [21]. Emotional disturbances secondary to prejudice and discrimination cause and are caused by obesity [32]. Overall, the obese have decreased mental health, general well-being, social interaction, functional capacity, and intellectual performance [33].

Socioeconomic class

An inverse relationship exists between social class and degree of obesity compared with controls [6]. This relationship is independent of parental class or level of education. Young obese females are less likely to be married, complete fewer years of school, and have lower household incomes than their normal-weight counterparts. Males are also less likely to be married [34]. Both sexes are less likely to be admitted to prestigious colleges [34a].

Weight discrimination at work leads to a decreased chance of being hired; this bias is greater toward women than men [35]. The weight-based discrimination occurs at every stage of the employment cycle: compensation, promotion, discipline and discharge [35a]. Workplace discrimination against the overweight is not forbidden by federal law as is discrimination based on sex, race, religion, or national origin. There is little recourse available to the obese worker who is a victim of discrimination.

Quality of life

The 36-item Short-Form Survey (SF-36) is often used to measure quality of life [36]. It measures eight domains: physical function, role limitations secondary to health problems, social function, bodily pain, general mental health, role limitations secondary to emotional problems, vitality, and general health perceptions. The SF-36 addresses some characteristics that already have been discussed and others that have not been considered. It gives a validated indication of the overall burden of suffering associated with obesity. Most reports have shown decreased quality of life in obese patients compared with the general population. In particular, decreased vitality, social and occupational impairment, and bodily pain are prevalent. Disturbances not generally contained in quality-of-life surveys are pathologic hunger, sexual impairment, excessive perspiration, urinary incontinence, and inability to clean oneself [33].

Fox and colleagues [37] profiled questionnaires completed by 1200 obese patients who had had bariatric surgery or who had decided to have bariatric surgery. The respondents expressed low self-esteem and high levels of humiliation. They experienced embarrassment dealing with public chairs, hallways, and aisles that were too small to accommodate them. They also experienced embarrassment because of difficulties with cleanliness and odor. When shopping for clothes or food or eating in restaurants, they received hostility and contempt from the public. The respondents felt socially isolated and limited in their mobility. They expressed hopelessness, helplessness, and dissatisfaction with life.

Assessment tests

No results from any instrument for measuring psychiatric or psychologic pathology have been found to correlate consistently with weight loss after bariatric surgery. This finding is somewhat surprising if the difference in weight-loss outcomes after surgical intervention is considered to depend on behavioral elements such as compliance with diet and exercise regimens. Either the instruments are not measuring an important behavioral characteristic or postsurgical genetic/biochemical/neuroendocrine changes that are not fully characterized are the overruling forces that dictate weight-loss outcome. It is also possible that outcome predictors such as regular exercise or high self-esteem are merely correlates for psychologic profiles typical of those subsets of patients who are successful in losing weight and maintaining weight loss after surgery.

The more common use of psychiatric or psychologic measuring instruments has been to identify patients for whom surgery may be contraindicated, to identify patients who may need psychiatric intervention or ongoing support perioperatively, or to compare psychologic status before and after surgery. The psychologic work-up for patients before bariatric surgery has yet to be standardized. Box 1 lists the tests commonly used in the preoperative work-up.

Box 1. Preoperative assessment tests

Psychiatric/psychologic status
Minnesota Multiphasic Personality Inventory
Beck Depression Inventory
Profile of Mood States
Symptom Check List-90-Revised
Millon Clinical Multiaxial Inventory-II
Structured Clinical Interview for DSM-IV
Multidimensional Health Locus of Control
Millon Behavioral Medicine Diagnostic
Rosenberg Self-esteem Scale
Drug Abuse Screening Test
Alcohol Use Disorder Test-core

Eating disorder/eating patterns
Binge Eating Scale
Three-Factor Eating Questionnaire
Eating Disorder Questionnaire
Body Parts Satisfaction Questionnaire
Bulimia Cognitive Distortion Scale
Eating Disorder Examination
Eating Attitudes Test
Eating Disorder Index
Questionnaire on Weight and Eating Patterns-Revised
Emotional Eating Scales

Quality of life
36-item Short Form Health Status Survey
Lancashire Quality of Life Profile-European
Moorehead-Ardelt Quality of Life

The Veterans Affairs Administration has endorsed the use of five assessment tests in the preoperative work-up of bariatric patients within that system. The intent is to standardize and to collect data prospectively that may relate to outcome. The tests chosen to be used are Alcohol Use Disorder Test-core, Drug Abuse Screening Test, Millon Behavioral Medicine Diagnostic, Multidimensional Health Locus of Control, Questionnaire on Weight and Eating Patterns, and Minnesota Multiphasic Personality Inventory (MMPI).

Benefits of bariatric surgery by assessment test

The following are examples of assessment tests used to determine relationships of preoperative states and psychosocial or weight loss benefits after bariatric surgery: The MMPI scores were used to compare patients before and after gastric bypass [38]. MMPI profiles improved in 50% of patients. The 30% of patients with normal profiles preoperatively remained the same postoperatively. Patients who experienced major psychologic complications (15%) were a subset of the 20% who exhibited increased psychopathology postoperatively. MMPI-2 (revised MMPI) scores were analyzed as outcome predictors in 52 patients after gastric bypass [4]. Patients who lost less than 50% excess body weight loss (EBWL) scored significantly higher than the group that lost more than 50% EBWL on five scales that represent degree of reactivity to stress, potential for psycho-physiologic symptoms, emotional sensitivity, responsiveness to others' opinions, worry about health, and somatic complaints. The authors concluded that patients who were tense, anxious, and had excessive health concerns did not lose as much weight.

Measurements of 44 patients given the Diagnostic Interview Schedule and the Personality Diagnostic Questionnaire showed no or did not show a relationship between psychiatric disorders (axis I and II; *Diagnostic and Statistical Manual III* [DSM-III]) and weight loss 6 months after gastro-plasty [39]. In 130 patients who had bariatric surgery, preoperative psychiatric disorders (axis I and II; DSM-IV) showed no relationship to weight loss at follow-up 5.7 years after surgery [40]. Preoperative assessment of 77 patients by use of a semi-structured psychiatric interview yielded no predictive value for psychosocial variables of weight loss at 1, 2, or 3 years postoperatively [41].

The use of the Eating Disorder Inventory (EDI) in biliopancreatic diversion patients at 1 year after surgery showed increased psychologic benefit secondary to not having to diet and having a normal weight. This benefit was apparent only in patients who had not been preoccupied with their weight preoperatively, as determined by EDI score. Patients who were preoccupied by their weight before surgery continued to experience body dissatisfaction despite weight loss [21]. Patients undergoing gastric bypass and gastric banding may not incur such benefits, because losing weight without dieting is a consequence only of the less-often-performed biliopancreatic diversion procedure. When the EDI was given to 100 patients before vertical banded gastroplasty, it showed weight loss outcome to be positively correlated with the subscales measuring low body satisfaction, high drive for thinness, and low global scores [42].

Quality of life, however measured, is unanimously impaired preopera-tively and improved postoperatively [33]. Most obese patients consider impaired quality of life the most crippling aspect of their disease, and after surgery patients consider enhanced quality of life the greatest benefit [43]. Most patients undergoing bariatric surgery experience enhanced quality of life postoperatively with regard to psychosocial variables, psychiatric comorbidities, social functioning, self-esteem, and economic variables [42,44,45]. All of these outcomes are related to weight loss. A minority of patients (up to 30%) begin to regain weight at 18 months after bariatric procedure [18,40,46,47]. Reasons for this weight gain have not been fully characterized. Alternatively, one study showed decline in mood and depression gains 2 to 3 years after bariatric surgery despite excellent weight loss [48,49]. Negative quality-of-life outcomes remain atypical.

Predictors of weight loss

A systemic review of all psychiatric and psychosocial predictors of weight loss trialed in the last 20 years was recently conducted [51]. Significant findings were that psychiatric diagnoses, in general, predicted quality-of-life outcomes better than weight loss. Severe or chronic psychiatric diagnoses requiring inpatient hospitalization were related only to increased medical complications or poorer mental health outcomes. Depressive or anxiety symptoms as correlates of psychologic stress may be positive predictors of postoperative weight loss, particularly when the depression or anxiety is attributed directly to obesity. Personality disorders and personality traits had no predictive value.

Individual factors and their negative, positive, or lack of predictive value for weight-loss outcome after bariatric surgery are summarized in Table 1 and in Box 2. The factors listed have been tested as weight-loss correlates in at least one study, at a minimum of 1 year after surgery. Again, studies have shown conflicting results as exemplified by factors that seem to be negative and positive predictors and nonpredictors, as well (ie, eating sweets).

Existing challenges

It has been suggested that patients with certain eating patterns are better suited to certain bariatric procedures. Sweet-eaters may be served better by gastric bypass than by pure restricted procedures because an external constraint on eating refined sugar foods is imposed by the dumping syndrome [46]. Biliopancreatic diversion may assist binge eaters more effectively, because weight loss will occur whether or not the underlying food disorder resolves. Insufficient data exist at this time to endorse pathology-specific bariatric procedures.

In characterizing obese patients or analyzing them to predict surgical weight loss outcome, it must be remembered that surgical candidates have already been subjected to heavy selection bias. Surgical candidates are motivated to solve their weight problems. Most are from a socioeconomic group that has private health insurance and a support system that will foster success postoperatively. The Swedish Obese Subject studies found surgical patients to be more impaired than nonsurgical patients, as compared with matched controls [51]. Much of the research generated to date has been from specialized centers, many with multidisciplinary provider teams. Outcomes may not be representative of patients undergoing bariatric surgery in private practice or community settings [5].

Table 1
Negative and positive predictors of weight loss outcome after gastric bypass or gastric restrictive surgery

	Negative predictors	Positive predictors
Psychiatric/psychologic factors	Severe psychologic problems	Higher levels of psychologic stress
	Generalized anxiety	Increased phobia scores
	Acute depression	High self-esteem
	Psychosocial crisis	Marital dissatisfaction
	Suicidal ideation	Realization (preoperatively) that overeating was the cause of obesity
	Binge eating disorder or redevelopment of binge eating disorder	Feeling personally responsible for weight control
	Increased extrapunitiveness	
	Personality disorder	
Eating patterns/behavioral factors	High-calorie liquid or soft food consumption	Eating in response to sense of accomplishment
	Drinking carbonated beverages	Eating in response to pleasant feelings
	Sweet-eating behavior	Moderate alcohol consumption
	Nonsweet-eating behavior	Low food contacts
	Lack of exercise	Drinking water
	Eating poorly balanced meals or grazing and snacking	Eating three balanced meals and two snacks daily
		Regular exercise
		Sleeping seven hours per night
		Taking multivitamins, iron, and calcium
Demographic/biologic factors	Older age	Younger age
	Increased body mass index	Ody mass index <50
	Poor physical ability	Higher initial weight
	African American ethnicity	
	Diabetes mellitus	

Data from Herpertz S, Kielmann R, et al. Do psychosocial variables predict weight loss or mental health after obesity surgery? A systematic review. Obes Res 2004;12(10):1554–69.

The genetic control of postsurgical weight loss is not understood fully. Microarray assay data have indicated that the expression of certain gene groups in the visceral fat of patients with hyperlipidemia may be predictive of weight loss after gastric bypass (C. Warden, unpublished data). Such gene expression needs to characterized for other subpopulations of obese patients to understand better just how much of weight-loss outcome is genetically driven. What is the contribution of psychologic and environmental factors that interact with genetic expression?

Box 2. Factors that have no correlation with weight loss after surgery

Psychiatric/psychologic factors
Psychiatric abnormality
Untreated axis I diagnosis
Multiple axis I diagnosis
Previous hospitalization for psychiatric disorder
Binge eating disorder or other eating pathology
Alcohol or drug abuse
Emotional problems
History of significant life events
Violent parents/spouse
Parental/spousal support for bariatric surgery
Interpersonal behavior
Personality traits
High level of optimism
Intelligence

Eating patterns/behavioral factors
Success or effect of preoperative dieting
Presurgical eating behavior
Sweet eating or non-sweet eating

Demographic/biologic factors
Age
Age of onset of obesity
Family history of obesity
Gender
Ethnicity
Marital status
Weight at time of marriage
Unemployment
Socioeconomic status
Medical history
Diabetes mellitus

Data from Herpertz S, Kielmann R, et al. Do psychosocial variables predict weight loss or mental health after obesity surgery? A systematic review. Obes Res 2004;12(10):1554–69.

The biochemical mechanisms of weight loss after bariatric surgery are being actively studied. Ghrelin levels have been shown to be decreased for 6 months after gastric bypass and explain, in part, the anorexia that many patients experience [52,53]. Other neuroendocrine factors that play a role in satiety, weight set points, and metabolism require further clarification in patients who have had bariatric surgery to elucidate the underlying physiology. Genetics and metabolism may prove obese patients correct, who, when confronted with their inability to lose sufficient weight after surgery, say, "But it is not my fault!"

The belief that presurgical psychopathology predicts weight-loss outcome after bariatric surgery is not validated and is plagued by inconsistent evidence. Psychologic comorbidities do help estimate physical and mental well-being after bariatric surgery [54]. The statement that presurgical psychology does not predict weight-loss outcome may be premature, however. Instead of individual diagnoses predicting weight-loss outcome, it may be a certain profile or combination of psychosocial factors that is predictive. Certain personality traits together with a particular eating pattern in a certain setting of socioeconomic structure and psychologic history may predict accurately which patients will lose weight successfully. The notion that food or exercise behaviors alone are the factors that lead to successful weight loss and weight loss maintenance after surgery deserves further research. The relationships between eating behavior, energy intake and consumption, motivational systems, and psychologic function after bariatric surgery are not fully known [18,50].

Difficulties exist in generating needed research. It is no longer ethical to assign patients randomly to medical and surgical interventions in obesity treatment. The superior results of surgical intervention disallow such research. Comparative studies may be conducted while patients are undergoing medically supervised weight loss to meet criteria for bariatric surgery. Unfortunately, medical intervention studies have high dropout rates that weaken that arm of the study. While waiting for surgery, patients are exposed to the risks of continued comorbidities and possible worsening of disease [55]. Prospective observational studies designed with sufficient power to determine optimal amounts and rates of weight loss may be equivalent to randomized, controlled trials [56].

The use of preoperative patients as the control group for postoperative patients is flawed. A control group of successfully dieting patients would presumably show greater outcome differences. Patients undergoing weight loss from medical interventions show depression, anxiety, irritability, and preoccupation with food [57,58]. Patients losing weight by surgical intervention report enhanced positive emotions such as joy, increased self-confidence, and near effortless changes in eating habits [59].

Role of psychiatrists and psychologists

Are psychiatrists and psychologists essential in the preoperative work-up of candidates for bariatric surgery? They assess the patient's motivation and the presence of psychopathology. They provide education about the process of surgery and its behavioral challenges [5]. Most obese patients have unrealistic weight-loss expectations for bariatric surgery. Mental health professionals provide a forum to address these unrealistic expectations. A problematic axis I diagnosis, once unearthed, can be treated perioperatively and need not pose a contraindication to surgery. Nearly every axis I diagnosis has borne a surgical success reported in the literature; however, cooperation and compliance need to be assured within these diagnoses. Emotional disturbance has been shown retrospectively to complicate the postoperative course. Finally, patients must be declared competent to undergo informed consent.

Behavioral assessments of surgical candidates are conducted by nutritionists and psychologists. Along with psychologic testing, eating habits, exercise habits, weight history, and dieting history are elicited. A history of failed weight loss trials, often under medical supervision, is usually required for third-party reimbursement. Education concerning the postoperative diet and the necessary changes compared with the current diet is essential. A common example is the large intake of high-calorie, high-carbohydrate, carbonated beverages, which are not appropriate after bariatric surgery. Behavioral tenets that apply to successful weight loss and weight-loss maintenance in medical interventions largely apply to surgical patients as well [24,60]. Regular exercise correlates with maintenance of weight loss and enhanced lean body mass. Emotional cues and social situations related to overeating will still be in effect. It is helpful to problem solve and institute behavioral change before surgery to ease the transition postoperatively. The difference is that, in most patients after surgery, these behaviors result in significant and long-term weight loss because they are aided by early satiety and, in the case of gastric bypass, a period of anorexia.

The timing of surgical intervention may also be addressed by psychiatrists and psychologists. High environmental stress and lack of support in a patient's immediate environment have been correlated with poorer weight-loss outcome. Time off from work, time to shop for and prepare foods for the postoperative diet, and time for exercise must be accommodated.

References

[1] Wadden TA, Stunkard AJ. Social and psychological consequences of obesity. Ann Intern Med 1985;103(6 Pt 2):1062–7.
[2] Moore ME, Stunkard A, Srole L. Obesity, social class, and mental illness. JAMA 1962;181: 962–6.
[3] Crisp AH, McGuiness B. Jolly fat: relation between obesity and psychoneurosis in general population. BMJ 1976;1(6000):7–9.
[4] Tsushima WT, Bridenstine MP, Balfour JF. MMPI-2 scores in the outcome prediction of gastric bypass surgery. Obes Surg 2004;14(4):528–32.
[5] Stunkard AJ, Stinnett JL, Smoller JW. Psychological and social aspects of the surgical treatment of obesity. Am J Psychiatry 1986;143(4):417–29.

[6] Sonne-Holm S, Sorensen TI. Prospective study of attainment of social class of severely obese subjects in relation to parental social class, intelligence, and education. BMJ (Clin Res Ed) 1986;292(6520):586–9.

[7] Rand CS, Macgregor AM. Morbidly obese patients' perceptions of social discrimination before and after surgery for obesity. South Med J 1990;83(12):1390–5.

[8] Stunkard AJ, Wadden TA. Psychological aspects of severe obesity. Am J Clin Nutr 1992; 55(2 Suppl):524S–32S.

[9] Kaminsky J, Gadaleta D. A study of discrimination within the medical community as viewed by obese patients. Obes Surg 2002;12(1):14–8.

[10] Fitzgibbon ML, Stolley MR, Kirschenbaum DS. Obese people who seek treatment have different characteristics than those who do not seek treatment. Health Psychol 1993;12(5): 342–5.

[11] Dixon JB, Dixon ME, O'Brien PE. Depression in association with severe obesity: changes with weight loss. Arch Intern Med 2003;163(17):2058–65.

[12] Kodama K, Noda S, Murakami A, et al. Depressive disorders as psychiatric complications after obesity surgery. Psychiatry Clin Neurosci 1998;52(5):471–6.

[13] Gertler R, Ramsey-Stewart G. Pre-operative psychiatric assessment of patients presenting for gastric bariatric surgery (surgical control of morbid obesity). Aust N Z J Surg 1986; 56(2):157–61.

[14] Balsiger BM, Murr MM, Poggio JL, et al. Bariatric surgery. Surgery for weight control in patients with morbid obesity. Med Clin North Am 2000;84(2):477–89.

[15] Black DW, Goldstein RB, Mason EE. Prevalence of mental disorder in 88 morbidly obese bariatric clinic patients. Am J Psychiatry 1992;149(2):227–34.

[16] Wooley SC, Garner DM. Obesity treatment: the high cost of false hope. J Am Diet Assoc 1991;91(10):1248–51.

[17] Carpenter KM, Hasin DS, Allison DB, et al. Relationships between obesity and DSM-IV major depressive disorder, suicide ideation, and suicide attempts: results from a general population study. Am J Public Health 2000;90(2):251–7.

[18] Hsu LK, Benotti PN, Dwyer J, et al. Nonsurgical factors that influence the outcome of bariatric surgery: a review. Psychosom Med 1998;60(3):338–46.

[19] Hsu LK. Epidemiology of the eating disorders. Psychiatr Clin North Am 1996;19(4): 681–700.

[20] Powers PS, Perez A, Boyd F, et al. Eating pathology before and after bariatric surgery: a prospective study. Int J Eat Disord 1999;25(3):293–300.

[21] Adami GF, Gandolfo P, Campostano A, et al. Eating disorder inventory in the assessment of psychosocial status in the obese patients prior to and at long-term following biliopancreatic diversion for obesity. Int J Eat Disord 1994;15(3):265–74.

[22] Kissileff HR. Is there an eating disorder in the obese? Ann N Y Acad Sci 1989;575:410–9 [discussion: 424–30].

[23] Delin CR, Watts JM, Saebel JL, et al. An exploration of the outcomes of gastric bypass surgery for morbid obesity: patient characteristics and indices of success. Obes Surg 1995; 5(2):159–70.

[24] Cook CM, Edwards C. Success habits of long-term gastric bypass patients. Obes Surg 1999; 9(1):80–2.

[25] Adami GF, Gandolfo P, Dapueto R, et al. Eating behavior following biliopancreatic diversion for obesity: study with a three-factor eating questionnaire. Int J Eat Disord 1993; 14(1):81–6.

[26] Stunkard AJ. The dieting depression; incidence and clinical characteristics of untoward responses to weight reduction regimens. Am J Med 1957;23(1):77–86.

[27] Adami GF, Meneghelli A, Scopinaro N. Night eating and binge eating disorder in obese patients. Int J Eat Disord 1999;25(3):335–8.

[28] Latner JD, Wetzler S, Goodman ER, et al. Gastric bypass in a low-income, inner-city population: eating disturbances and weight loss. Obes Res 2004;12(6):956–61.

[29] Stunkard AJ, Grace WJ, Wolff HG. The night-eating syndrome; a pattern of food intake among certain obese patients. Am J Med 1955;19(1):78–86.

[30] Brosin HW. The psychiatric aspects of obesity. JAMA 1954;155(14):1238–9.

[31] Stunkard AJ, Sorensen TI. Obesity and socioeconomic status–a complex relation. N Engl J Med 1993;329(14):1036–7.

[32] Mills JK. A note on interpersonal sensitivity and psychotic symptomatology in obese adult outpatients with a history of childhood obesity. J Psychol 1995;129(3):345–8.

[33] Kral JG, Sjostrom LV, Sullivan MB. Assessment of quality of life before and after surgery for severe obesity. Am J Clin Nutr 1992;55(2 Suppl):611S–4S.

[34] Gortmaker SL, Must A, Perrin JM, et al. Social and economic consequences of overweight in adolescence and young adulthood. N Engl J Med 1993;329(14):1008–12.

[34a] Canning H, Mayer J. Obesity: its possible effect on college acceptance. The New England Journal of Medicine 1966;275(21):1172–4.

[35] Roe DA, Eickwort KR. Relationships between obesity and associated health factors with unemployment among low income women. J Am Med Womens Assoc 1976;31(5):193–4 198–9; 203–4.

[35a] Roehling MV. Weight based discrimination in employment: psychological and legal aspects. Personnel Psychology 1999;52:969–1016.

[36] Ware JE Jr, Sherbourne CD. The MOS 36-item short-form health survey (SF-36). I. Conceptual framework and item selection. Med Care 1992;30(6):473–83.

[37] Fox KM, Taylor SL, et al. Understanding the bariatric surgical patient: a demographic, lifestyle and psychological profile. Obes Surg 2000;10(5):477–81.

[38] Saltzstein EC, Gutmann MC. Gastric bypass for morbid obesity: preoperative and postoperative psychological evaluation of patients. Arch Surg 1980;115(1):21–8.

[39] Black DW, Goldstein RB, Mason EE. Psychiatric diagnosis and weight loss following gastric surgery for obesity. Obes Surg 2003;13(5):746–51.

[40] Powers PS, Rosemurgy A, Boyd F, et al. Outcome of gastric restriction procedures: weight, psychiatric diagnoses, and satisfaction. Obes Surg 1997;7(6):471–7.

[41] Schrader G, Stefanovic S, Gibbs A, et al. Do psychosocial factors predict weight loss following gastric surgery for obesity? Aust N Z J Psychiatry 1990;24(4):496–9.

[42] Guisado JA, Vaz FJ, Alarcon J, et al. Psychopathological status and interpersonal functioning following weight loss in morbidly obese patients undergoing bariatric surgery. Obes Surg 2002;12(6):835–40.

[43] Buchwald H, Avidor Y, Braunwald E, et al. Bariatric surgery: a systematic review and meta-analysis. JAMA 2004;292(14):1724–37.

[44] Solow C. Psychosocial aspects of intestinal bypass surgery for massive obesity: current status. Am J Clin Nutr 1977;30(1):103–8.

[45] Herpertz S, Kielmann R, Wolf AM, et al. Does obesity surgery improve psychosocial functioning? A systematic review. Int J Obes Relat Metab Disord 2003;27(11):1300–14.

[46] Sugerman HJ, Starkey JV, Birkenhauer R, et al. A randomized prospective trial of gastric bypass versus vertical banded gastroplasty for morbid obesity and their effects on sweets versus non-sweets eaters. Ann Surg 1987;205(6):613–24.

[47] Pories WJ, Swanson MS, MacDonald KG. Who would have thought it? An operation proves to be the most effective therapy for adult-onset diabetes mellitus. Ann Surg 1995; 222(3):339–50 [discussion: 350–2].

[48] Waters GS, Pories WJ, Swanson MS, et al. Long-term studies of mental health after the Greenville gastric bypass operation for morbid obesity. Am J Surg 1991;161(1):154–7 [discussion: 157–8].

[49] Karlsson J, Sjostrom L, Sullivan M. Swedish obese subjects (SOS)—an intervention study of obesity. Two-year follow-up of health-related quality of life (HRQL) and eating behavior after gastric surgery for severe obesity. Int J Obes Relat Metab Disord 1998;22(2):113–26.

[50] Herpertz S, Kielmann R, Wolf AM. Do psychosocial variables predict weight loss or mental health after obesity surgery? A systematic review. Obes Res 2004;12(10):1554–69.

[51] Kral JG, Heymsfield S. Morbid obesity: definitions, epidemiology, and methodological problems. Gastroenterol Clin North Am 1987;16(2):197–205.

[52] Halverson JD, Koehler RE. Gastric bypass: analysis of weight loss and factors determining success. Surgery 1981;90(3):446–55.

[53] Delin CR, Watts JM, Bassett DL. An exploration of the outcomes of gastric bypass surgery for morbid obesity: patient characteristics and indeces of success. Obes Surg 1995;5(2): 159–70.

[54] Valley V, Grace DM. Psychosocial risk factors in gastric surgery for obesity: identifying guidelines for screening. Int J Obes 1987;11(2):105–13.

[55] Kral JG. Selection of patients for anti-obesity surgery. Int J Obes Relat Metab Disord 2001; 25(Suppl 1):S107–12.

[56] Benson K, Hartz AJ. A comparison of observational studies and randomized, controlled trials. N Engl J Med 2000;342(25):1878–86.

[57] Halmi KA, Stunkard AJ, Mason EE. Emotional responses to weight reduction by three methods: gastric bypass, jejunoileal bypass, diet. Am J Clin Nutr 1980;33(2 Suppl):446–51.

[58] Andersen T, Backer OG, Stokholm KH, et al. Randomized trial of diet and gastroplasty compared with diet alone in morbid obesity. N Engl J Med 1984;310(6):352–6.

[59] Mills MJ, Stunkard AJ. Behavioral changes following surgery for obesity. Am J Psychiatry 1976;133(5):527–31.

[60] Bull RH, Engels WD, Engelsmann F, et al. Behavioural changes following gastric surgery for morbid obesity: a prospective, controlled study. J Psychosom Res 1983;27(6):457–67.

ELSEVIER
SAUNDERS

SURGICAL
CLINICS OF
NORTH AMERICA

Surg Clin N Am 85 (2005) 757–771

Quality Assurance in Bariatric Surgery

Stewart E. Rendon, MD*, Walter J. Pories, MD

*Division of Bariatric Surgery, Brody School of Medicine at East Carolina University,
600 Moye Boulevard, Greenville, NC 27834, USA*

The numbers are staggering. Morbid obesity, the most severe form, afflicts more 23 million Americans with a body mass index (BMI = Wt [kg]/ Ht[M]^2) of 35 or higher (ie, who exceed their ideal body weight by about 100 pounds) [1]. Eight million Americans have a BMI of 40 or higher. Of even greater concern is the increasing prevalence of morbid obesity among the young. In the United States, more than 10% of children ages 2 to 5 years are now overweight, an increase from 7% in 1994 [2]. In some cohorts of the United States population, 5% of the children are affected. Approximately 1 million youths between the ages of 12 and 19 years have the metabolic syndrome. With an increase of 33% during the last decade, obesity will probably overtake tobacco use as the leading preventable cause of mortality by 2010.

Bulk, as limiting as it is, is not the most serious problem for the morbidly obese. Severe obesity is associated with serious comorbidities, including diabetes, hypertension, Pickwickian syndrome, cardiopulmonary failure, sleep apnea, crippling arthritis, pseudotumor cerebri, polycystic ovary syndrome, infertility, stress incontinence, and gastroesophageal reflux disease, among others. Most severely obese persons have difficulty finding jobs; employers are aware of their high rates of absenteeism and their high health care costs. Perhaps because of their isolation and frequent instances of abuse, about 25% require formal psychiatric care. Premature deaths are common.

Bariatric surgery is still the only recommended treatment for severe obesity, a conclusion reached by the National Institutes of Health (NIH) Consensus Conference on the Surgery of Obesity in 1991, when it declared that traditional nonsurgical approaches are not effective in these individuals and that patients with a BMI of 40 or higher or a BMI of 35 or higher with

---

* Corresponding author.
E-mail address: drrendon@aol.com (S.E. Rendon).

0039-6109/05/$ - see front matter © 2005 Elsevier Inc. All rights reserved.
doi:10.1016/j.suc.2005.04.005

comorbidities are surgical candidates. Growth in bariatric surgery has been rapid: more than 120,000 procedures were performed in 2003, compared with fewer than 20,000 in 1993.

Bariatric surgery carries substantial risks, including death. The operations are technically challenging, the patients present with complex metabolic derangements, nursing care of these huge individuals is difficult, and there can be serious short- and long-term complications. With care, experience, and organization, however, some centers are able to report large series with minimal mortality and morbidity rates. Blackstone reported 700 consecutive cases without a death, and Wittgrove reported more than 2500 cases with only one death (Robin Blackstone, MD, and Alan Wittgrove, MD, personal communication, 2004).

Unfortunately, not all centers have equally good results. As the demand increased, surgeons with little experience or training in bariatric surgery streamed into the field, often with disastrous outcomes. Lawsuits quickly followed, as patients experienced leaks, sepsis, multiorgan failure, anastomotic stenoses, fistulas, dehiscences, and other multiple consequences of technical failures. More litigation was stimulated by the peculiar late complications of bariatric procedures including internal hernias, closed loop obstructions, staple-line breakdowns, and severe nutritional complications including full-blown pellagra, kwashiorkor, beriberi, and Wernicke–Korsakoff syndrome.

By 2003, a number of malpractice carriers refused to insure bariatric surgeons or set the premiums at unreachable levels. By 2004, several third-party payers, including Blue Cross Blue Shield of Florida and CIGNA Healthcare, as well as a number of HMOs, announced that they would no longer cover the surgery. Other carriers were prepared to follow suit.

A lack of access to care

These developments left bariatric surgeons and the American Society for Bariatric Surgery (ASBS) in a curious situation: there was a national epidemic, successful therapies were available, but the treatment could not be provided to those who needed it. With 120,000 cases per year being performed, bariatric surgery is available to less than 1% of those who could benefit from the procedures.

If there were a pill that could produce a durable weight loss of 100 lbs or more and induce full remission of diabetes, asthma, hypertension, sleep apnea, and stress incontinence while sharply ameliorating arthritis, allowing these sufferers to return to work, would the public accept a decision to limit the medicine to only 1% of those who could benefit?

On the other hand, the ASBS was in no position to promote the surgery if it could not be delivered safely and if it could not reassure the public that there were centers capable of providing the surgical care with efficacy, efficiency, and safety.

The American Society for Bariatric Surgery responds with four initiatives

To respond to the crisis, the leadership of the ASBS agreed that the American public deserved the assurance of quality bariatric surgery. To meet this challenge, the officers decided the best initial step was to re-examine the following issues:

1. What are the findings in the literature? Are the claims of success well founded? What are the real complication rates?
2. What are the best current practices?
3. How can research, especially protocols that examine the mechanisms reversed by bariatric surgery, be stimulated and supported?
4. How can continuous quality improvement methodologies be introduced into bariatric surgery?

Assessing the literature

A meta-analysis of the literature pertaining to bariatric surgery written in the English language was conducted under the direction of Buchwald [3]. This review of 2738 citations in the English language between 1990 and 2003 concluded that excess weight loss for all 22,094 patients reported was 61.2% (58.15–64.4%), 47.5% for gastric banding, 61.6% for gastric bypass, 68.2% for gastroplasty; and 70.1% for biliopancreatic or duodenal switch. Operative mortality (≤ 30 days) was 0.1% for restrictive procedures such as gastric banding, 0.5% for gastric bypass, and 1.1% for biliopancreatic diversion or duodenal switch. Diabetes was completely resolved in 61.7% of patients and resolved or improved in 86%. Hyperlipidemia improved in 70% or more patients. Hypertension was resolved in 61.7% of patients and resolved or improved in 78.5%. Obstructive sleep apnea was resolved in 85.7% of patients and improved in 83.6% of patients.

Assessment of best practices

To assess the best current practices, the ASBS held a Consensus Conference at Georgetown University, Washington, DC, on May 5 through 7, 2004, using the format that the NIH uses for such fact-finding sessions. The panel's report, to be published soon in the *Journal of the American College of Surgeons* agreed with the mega-analysis that

1. Bariatric surgery produces durable weight control.
2. Bariatric surgery is an effective therapy for the control of the comorbidities of morbid obesity.
3. In expert hands, bariatric surgery can be performed with minimal complications and low mortality rates.
4. Research is needed.

Research initiatives

The NIH, fully aware of the crisis and the promise of bariatric surgery, funded a $15 million program in bariatric surgical research entitled the Longitudinal Assessment of Bariatric Surgery (LABS). This program involves six national bariatric surgical centers: Columbia/Cornell, East Carolina University, the University of California at Davis, the University of North Dakota, the University of Pittsburgh, and the University of Washington. The specific aims of the LABS program include clinical research as well as basic science protocols that examine the mechanisms for the remarkable effects of bariatric surgery on obesity-associated comorbidities (eg, why does diabetes disappear before there is significant weight loss?). In addition to the LABS platform, additional substudies and ancillary studies are being funded to explore various aspects of the surgical advance. The website, http://win.niddk.nih.gov/publications/labs/labs804.pdf, offers additional details about the LABS project.

The introduction of continuous quality improvement methodology

Quality improvement

Quality improvement methods are essentially ways to bring a quality product to market, with efficacy, efficiency, and safety. Quality is improved by a cycle that defines the objective, establishes measures of quality, applies these standards to the production and delivery of the product, evaluates the outcomes, and, finally, improves quality by continuous learning from the process [4]. The Japanese revolutionized the worldwide automotive industry by creating and implementing this method [5]. The method is not new, but it has been used little in bariatric surgery [6,7].

The same method can be applied to establish quality in bariatric surgery. Although the use of the words "business" and "medicine" in the same sentence may appear pejorative, adopting "business" methods and ideas could help greatly in optimizing quality in bariatric surgery.

Defining quality

The quality of surgical care traditionally has been measured by process (ie, Are the surgeons certified? How many surgical beds are available and how are they staffed? Do the residents sign verbal orders in time? Are the charts completed in time?).

These measures no longer suffice. Employers and insurance carriers, those who pay the bills, now demand a new approach, the definition of quality by outcomes as defined by the stakeholders (patients, referring physicians, surgeons, third-party payers, bariatric community, and malpractice carriers). Measuring outcomes data enables comparisons of procedures by degree of weight loss, resolution of comorbidities, short- and long-term complications, improvement of quality of life, return to the activities of daily living, and employment. In short, quality is defined by objective and relevant measures.

Quality assurance

Quality assurance is the methodology by which the quality of a product is assured. If an appropriate quality assurance methodology can be applied to bariatric surgery, it will assure the public that the product is delivered regularly with efficacy (it works), with efficiency (conserving resources, including financial resources), and safely (with the minimum morbidity and mortality) [8].

Quality assurance focuses on producing confidence that quality requirements will be fulfilled. It must be exercised from the research and development stage, throughout production, testing, and postmarketing surveillance. The system of quality assurance must identify all process failures, control for variations, assess the capability of producing a product, analyze the times and causes of breakdowns in the process, and control improvement actions. These steps will help in obtaining remedial action before commencement of production [9]. Each of these processes can be applied to bariatric surgery with the same rigor now required for the production of pharmaceuticals and medical devices. Admittedly, the goal is difficult, but it is feasible.

Advance quality planning

Advance quality planning (AQP) is the process of planning in advance to reduce problems. The fundamentals of advance quality planning are essentially proper planning, preparation, and attention to detail. AQP is a reliable quality-assurance method used to achieve product quality and reliability. AQP significantly reduces risks caused by delays, optimizes costs, and provides products that perform with minimal variation [5].

Industrial failures are usually related to inadequate management and quality control rather than technology. The quality of a product must be planned, step by step. When too much time is wasted dealing with problems, production suffers, and management has to juggle resources.

AQP involves paying rigorous attention to detail in all areas of the design process, weeding out feasibility issues before production, and identifying potential process failures. AQP can be used internally and externally, to set standards for oneself and any suppliers.

Bariatric surgery has now progressed from the early stages of product development to a mature level where the public expects predictable outcomes delivered with a minimal expenditure of resources and maximum safety. Reliable operations now exist. If these procedures and the care paths are standardized, if outcomes are measured rigorously on all patients, and if records are maintained meticulously, bariatric surgery can be improved in a continuous process. Critics claim that these rigorous controls prevent progress, but those criticisms are incorrect: none of these approaches interferes with the development of new surgical approaches under institutional review board control.

Quality assurance managers

The quality assurance manager is responsible for the quality management system and monitors and advises on how the system is performing. The work of a quality assurance manager involves coordinating activities required to direct and control an organization with regard to quality. It often includes the publication of statistics regarding company performance against set parameters of quality [10]. In successful centers, the most senior bariatric surgeon, with strong support at the highest level of administration, usually serves as the quality assurance manager.

Application of industrial principles

As data accumulated showing that bariatric surgery is effective and can be delivered with remarkable efficacy, efficiency, and safety, surgeons became determined to improve the delivery systems for bariatric surgery. To accomplish this aim, the ASBS held multiple consultations with the various stakeholders in bariatric surgery, including industry, federal and state agencies, manufacturers, health insurance carriers, HMOs, professional liability carriers, bariatric surgeons in academia and in private practice, and several other professional societies. These discussions led to the formation of the Surgical Review Committee (SRC) based on the following conclusions:

1. Bariatric surgery is a major medical advance, able to produce durable weight loss and remarkable remissions of comorbidities.
2. Bariatric surgery and the care of morbidly obese patients is a demanding and complex specialty.
3. Although many centers deliver excellent bariatric surgical services, there are unacceptable and preventable differences in outcomes in perioperative mortality and morbidity.
4. Outcomes can be improved by comparing outcomes and care paths with a continuing quality improvement program that will clarify indications, compare procedures, and guide bariatric surgeons in perioperative and long-term care.
5. The process is most likely to succeed if it is initiated by the bariatric surgical community.
6. The process must be voluntary and appropriately rewarded.
7. The process must be fair and transparent with the ability to appeal decisions.
8. The process must be administered by an independent, not-for-profit organization.

9. The organization must include the various stakeholders in bariatric surgery.
10. The organization shall not determine what operations or care are to be followed at each center. Only the bariatric surgical teams at these institutions can make those determinations. Whatever choices are made, each center must agree to standardize them to yield reliable data to permit comparisons and quality improvement.
11. The process must be based on outcomes rather than process.
12. Data must be verified by site visits.

The proposal to implement the quality improvement initiative was adopted enthusiastically by the membership at the annual business meeting of the ASBS held in June 2003. Two amendments were defeated:

1. That centers be stratified into levels.
2. That surgeons with excellent outcomes be identified as master surgeons.

The first amendment was defeated by the argument that insurance carriers might choose to reward only level 1 centers. The second was defeated because the designation was deemed unnecessary and possibly pejorative to capable surgeons who, for one reason or another, did not qualify for the title.

The environment: an urgency to proceed

The actions of the ASBS did not occur in a vacuum. Several Blue Cross and Blue Shield carriers announced programs to identify Centers of Excellence, other carriers launched their own Institutes of Bariatric Surgical Excellence, and other companies developed individual contracts with surgeons or hospitals. These initiatives led to a confusion of standards with variations in work-up requirements, differences in indications, refusal to support operations already in wide use, and the denial of laparoscopic approaches because they were considered experimental by some payers.

The biggest concern, however, was the disparate collection of data by each of the entities. Without uniform definition of data elements, without standardization of procedures and care paths, without confirmation of the accuracy of the data, and without the ability to share the information, methodologies of continuous quality improvement could not be developed effectively and accurately. Under those conditions, everyone would lose—most of all the patients.

Therefore, the Executive Council of the ASBS agreed that an ASBS Centers of Excellence program should be developed as quickly as possible.

The Surgical Review Corporation

In accordance with the instructions of the Executive Council of the ASBS, three of its leaders, Champion, Pories, and Wittgrove, founded the

Surgical Review Corporation (SRC), a separate, nonprofit company, in November 2003 with the assistance of Michael Hartney, corporate legal counsel for the ASBS. Gary Pratt was hired to serve as the executive director. Pories was elected president, Wittgrove became vice-president, and Champion became secretary-treasurer.

The Board of Governors

The three officers then selected the Board of Governors to represent the major stakeholders in bariatric surgery (Table 1). The effort to include the American College of Surgeons is reflected by the choice of two former presidents and a former chair of the ACS Board of Governors.

Table 1
The Board of Governors of the Surgery Review Corporation

Name	Background	Member ASBS	Member ACS
Bart Bandy	CEO, Inamed (industry)		
Henry Buchwald	Bariatric surgeon, former President ASBS	X	X
Kenneth Champion	Bariatric surgeon	X	X
Michael Faber	Consumer		
Jennifer Giannos	Registered nurse		
Robert Greczyn	CEO, Blue Cross and Blue Shield of North Carolina		
Dale Jenkins	CEO, Medical Mutual Co. of North Carolina		
R. Scott Jonesa	Surgeon, employee of ACS and former President ACS		X
Kenneth MacWilliams	Former investment banker		
Patrick O'Leary[a]	Bariatric surgeon, former Chair of ACS Board of Governors, former president ASBS	X	X
Tracy Owens	RN, former President Allied Health, ASBS	X	
Walter Pories	Bariatric surgeon, former President ASBS	X	X
George Sheldona	Surgeon, former President ACS		X
Alan Wittgrove	Bariatric surgeon, former President ASBS	X	X
David Hunt[b]	Surgeon, Medicare administrator		X

Abbreviations: ACS, American College of Surgeons; ASBS, American Society for Bariatric Surgery.

[a] Although Jones, Sheldon, and O'Leary were chosen because of their leadership roles in the American College of Surgeons, they were not selected by the ACS, nor are they acting in an official capacity for that organization.

[b] Hunt is not a formal member of the Board of Governors because in his position with Medicare is unable to serve in an official capacity. He has been invited to participate as a permanent guest to keep the Board informed about Medicare and Medicaid interests.

The Bariatric Surgery Review Committee

The members of the Bariatric Surgery Review Committee, selected by the Board of Governors with the advice of the officers, are listed in Table 2. All are experienced bariatric surgeons, and all are members of the ASBS and the ACS. One third of the members are from the academic community; two thirds are from the private sector.

Requirements for recognition as an American Society for Bariatric Surgery Centers of Excellence

The requirements for recognition as an ASBS Center of Excellence were derived after multiple meetings among experienced bariatric surgeons with the advice of members of industry familiar with continuous quality improvement methodologies. The following basic principles were derived for the process:

1. Bariatric surgical care is a combined effort that involves a multidisciplinary team and a well-equipped facility.
2. Participation in the national quality improvement program is voluntary.
3. Centers are to be judged by outcomes rather than by process.
4. Data submitted in the applications are to be verified by site visits.

Table 2
Members of the Bariatric Surgery Review Committee

Name	Location	Academic post	Member of ASBS	Member of ACS
Robin Blackstone, MD, FACS	Scottsdale, AZ		X	X
Carlos Carrasquilla, MD, FACS	Fort Lauderdale, FL		X	X
Ken Champion, MD, FACS	Atlanta, GA		X	X
David Flum, MD, FACS	Seattle, WA	X	X	X
Sayeed Ikramuddin, MD, FACS	Minneapolis, MN	X	X	X
James Michael Kane, MD, FACS	Arlington Heights, IL		X	X
Kenneth MacDonald, MD, FACS	Greenville, NC	X	X	X
Blaine Neese, MD, FACS	Garden Grove, CA		X	X
Ninh Nguyen, MD, FACS	Orange, CA		X	X
Philip Schauer, MD, FACS	Cleveland, OH	X	X	X
Harvey Sugerman, MD, FACS[a]	Sanibel Isle, FL	X	X	X
Donald Waldrep, MD, FACS	Roseville, CA		X	X

Abbreviations: ACS, American College of Surgeons; ASBS, American Society for Bariatric Surgery.

[a] Since the election, Sugerman resigned because of a potential conflict of interest with his position as president of the ASBS; Hutcher, the president-elect of the ASBS, will serve in his place until the annual meeting of the ASBS. At that time, Hutcher will resign, and it is possible that the Board of Governors will restore Sugerman's position on the Committee. Additional appointments to the Review Committee are expected to provide a broader base to perform the reviews.

The Centers of Excellence application process

The application process was divided into two steps:

1. Provisional status requires documentation that the applicants (ie, the individual surgeons, the surgical group, and the hospitals) have the resources to deliver optimal bariatric surgical services.
2. Full approval requires documentation that the applicants have a record of excellent short- and long-term outcomes in bariatric surgery.

There are several advantages to this two-step approach. The application for provisional status is designed to allow candidates to determine whether they want to make the investment to deliver bariatric surgical services, to guide hospitals and surgeons in the development of bariatric surgical centers, and, to discourage marginal centers from staying in the field. The granting of provisional status is a private designation that cannot be released to the public (ie, used for advertising or other purposes). Achievement of provisional status leads to an invitation to submit an application for full approval, a complex process that requires the submission of short- and long-term data that are verified by a site visit.

Both sets of applications are reviewed initially and independently by two members of the Review Committee. Reviewers are tentatively selected by SRC staff to review an application. Review Committee members use a process before reviewing an application to determine whether they have a conflict of interest. If no conflict of interest exists, the two reviewers examine the application independently and provide summaries to the full Committee for final decisions. An appeals process for rejected applicants to the Board of Governors is in place.

The SRC does not certify or accredit centers but instead is under contract with the ASBS to administer its program independently. The recognition as an ASBS Center of Excellence is granted by the Society upon notification by the SRC that the required standards have been met.

Requirements for provisional status

There are 11 requirements for provisional status.

1. There is an institutional commitment at the highest levels of the applicant medical staff and the institution's administration to excellence in the care of bariatric surgical patients as documented with an ongoing regularly scheduled in-service education program in bariatric surgery.

This requirement refers to a culture in which the staff is prepared to manage morbidly obese patients with understanding and compassion and to appreciate the burdens of the comorbidities of the disease. The staff should be aware of the basic concepts of bariatric surgery through in-service programs. Those directly caring for these patients should be able to recognize the early signs of the common complications, including pulmonary embolus, anastomotic leak, infection, and bowel obstruction, so that these complications can be managed promptly.

2. The applicant institution has performed at least 125 bariatric surgical cases in the preceding 12 months, and each applicant surgeon has performed at least 125 total bariatric cases and performed at least 50 cases in the preceding 12 months.

Bariatric surgical cases are defined as primary operations (as listed in Question 9 of the Procedure Preferences of the Provisional Status Application), emergency procedures, or revisions. Endoscopies, placement of feeding jejunostomies, hernia repairs, and plastic surgical reconstructions are not included in this classification.

3. The applicant maintains a Medical Director for bariatric surgery who participates in the relevant decision-making administrative meetings of the institution.

The position of Medical Director shall be filled by a qualified bariatric surgeon who is appointed through the administrative/medical staff process with hospital minutes documenting his or her participation in the bariatric program decisions. Regularly scheduled meetings to address the bariatric program in the institution that involve medical staff, nursing, administration, central supply, operating room personnel, and the business office are required.

4. The applicant maintains a full complement of the various consultative services required for the care of bariatric surgical patients including the immediate availability of full in-house critical care services.

This requirement includes the availability of, at the least, an anesthesiologist, a pulmonologist, a cardiologist, an interventional radiologist, and an infectious disease specialist, plus nutritional and psychology/psychiatry support. The facility must have an ICU that has a full-time staff with experience managing critically ill morbidly obese patients with ventilators and invasive hemodynamic monitoring technologies. An outpatient surgical center does not qualify as a bariatric surgical Center of Excellence.

5. The applicant maintains a full line of equipment and instruments for the care of bariatric surgical patients including furniture, wheel chairs, operating room tables, beds, radiologic facilities, surgical instruments, and other facilities suitable for morbidly obese and superobese patients.

Furniture, beds, scales, wheel chairs, operating room tables and litters, strong enough and extra wide to accommodate the severely obese at the weight limits established by the institution, must be available for patients who need this specialized equipment. Patient movement/transfer systems for morbidly obese patients must be in place throughout the institution wherever the morbidly obese receive care. CT scans with sufficient capacity to handle morbidly obese patients and the ability to perform Gastrografin swallows and nuclear medicine scans are essential. Ambulances serving the institution should also be equipped to manage these large patients with appropriate stretchers, straps, and transfer devices. Finally, and perhaps most important, the staff must be trained to use the equipment and be capable of moving these large individuals without injury either to the patients or the staff.

6. The applicant has a bariatric surgeon who spends a significant portion of his or her efforts in the field of bariatric surgery and who has qualified coverage and support for patient care.

The surgeon must be certified by the American Board of Surgery or an equivalent board recognized by the Accreditation Committee for Graduate Medical Education (ACGME). In addition, the surgeon must show evidence of bariatric surgical expertise in accordance with the guidelines of the ASBS.

Qualified coverage is defined as the coverage required for the full care of a bariatric patient in the absence of the primary surgeon. The covering surgeon should be certified by the American Board of Surgery, have significant experience in the care of bariatric surgical patients, and be capable of managing the full range of complications associated with surgery of the morbidly obese.

7. The applicant uses clinical pathway orders that facilitate the standardization of perioperative care for the relevant procedure. In addition, all bariatric surgical procedures are standardized for each surgeon.

It is the surgeon's responsibility to select the primary operations he or she will perform and it is the expectation of the SRC that the procedures, no matter what the choice, will be done in a standardized manner. Similarly, the surgeon should determine the details of the planned perioperative care. These details will be documented so that each member of the surgeon's team is aware of the care plan and is prepared to follow the process as outlined by the surgeon. Unless such a process is followed, outcomes cannot be evaluated.

8. The applicant uses designated nurses or physician extenders who are dedicated to serving bariatric surgical patients and who are involved in continuing education in the care of bariatric patients.

The hospital should have a subset of nurses who routinely care for the bariatric patients and receive regular in-service education on their care, preferably assigned to a designated bariatric floor or wing. A bariatric coordinator should be designated to supervise the bariatric program.

The physician's practice should also have nursing and physician extenders who provide continuing education and care to the bariatric patients in the practice. This staffing should be outlined in the practice policy if it is a split practice that still performs significant general surgery.

9. The applicant makes available organized and supervised support groups for all patients who have undergone bariatric surgery at the institution.

The activities of the support group should be documented, including group locations, meeting times, supervisor, curriculum, and attendance. For example, such activities as on-line chat rooms, web-based support groups, exercise, instruction, and clothing sales should be noted.

10. The applicant provides documentation of a program dedicated to a goal of long-term patient follow-up of at least 75% for bariatric procedures at 5 years with a monitoring and tracking system for outcomes and agrees to provide annual outcome summaries to the SRC in a manner consistent with Health Insurance Portability and Accountability Act of 1996 (HIPAA) regulations.

This requirement is based on the observation that a significant number of patients develop nutritional deficiencies, internal and external hernias, return of previous emotional disorders, and other late complications. There is no requirement that the surgeon provide the follow-up personally, only that he or she be aware of the long-term status of the patient. Accordingly, the follow-up data can be gathered during group sessions, reunions, or through visits at other physicians' offices.

11. The applicant agrees to enter all patients who undergo surgery in the group's or individual practice; no patients will be excluded.

The SRC will develop a template for the recommended database. The SRC will not recommend or require any specific software program but plans to provide a web-based instrument for surgeons who have not yet settled on an approach to maintain the required information.

Application for full approval

The application for full approval includes the same questions but also requests specific data regarding percentage of follow-up, surgical outcomes in terms of weight loss, change in BMI, resolution of comorbidities, perioperative and long-term mortalities, reoperations, readmissions, revisions, and academic activities. Copies of the application forms are available at www.surgicalreview.org.

Status of the program

This article is being written in December 2004, about 6 months before the naming of the first ASBS Centers of Excellence and perhaps a year before this article goes into print. It is difficult to predict the course of this grand experiment to improve bariatric surgery with the quality improvement tools used in industry. At this time, the signs of success are encouraging, with applications from 340 hospitals and more than 700 surgeons. Also encouraging is the response of the insurance carriers who have promised improved reimbursement, preferential referral, relief from prior approval, and lower malpractice premiums. Only time will tell how successful this effort will be.

The goal is to name the first-round applicants recognized for full approval as ASBS Centers of Excellence at the Society's annual meeting in June 2005. Accordingly, potential applicants were notified that they needed to meet a deadline of October 31, 2004, to allow adequate time for review of the applications for provisional status, invitation to submit applications for full approval, site visits, final review by the Committee, and the recommendation to the Executive Council of the ASBS. More than 300 applications from hospitals representing more than 700 surgeon coapplicants were received before the deadline. These applications are now being processed by the staff and the Review Committee.

Significance

This pilot program provides a cooperative platform on which the numerous stakeholders can develop a cooperative approach to the quality control and improvement in bariatric surgery. The creation of a central database consisting of 30,000 to 50,000 cases per year with outcomes from all sectors of the surgical community verified by site visits will facilitate the definition of indications and allow comparison of procedures, care paths, and outcomes. In addition, there is a promising initiative to develop this database with definitions that allow comparisons with The National Surgical Quality Improvement Program (NSQIP) and LABS. If that effort succeeds, it will provide a model for surgical databases supporting clinical, basic science, and public policy research. This information will be vital to the improvement in efficacy, efficiency, and safety of bariatric surgery.

If the plan succeeds, the benefits will be substantial. On this fiftieth anniversary of bariatric surgery, there is still uncertainty about the indications, the choices of operations, and the long-term outcomes. What are the risks in a 650-pound male? What is the role of bariatric surgery in pediatric obesity? Should a diabetic patient with a BMI of 32 be considered for a gastric bypass? Adequate data can improve the delivery of surgical services—no one, patients or surgeons or hospitals or carriers, benefits from the wrong operation or from complications. SRC offers the benefits of a centralized organization. Providers are tired of filling out applications for the numerous Centers of Excellence programs that are emerging.

Carriers will also benefit substantially. Bariatric quality control programs are expensive and disruptive. The SRC charges participants to cover costs where most payers cannot. The SRC performs the site visits, sparing the carriers from incurring staffing and other associated costs necessary to confirm the data received from participants.

The biggest benefit, of course, will be to patients. It will be interesting to read this article 1 year from now.

References

[1] Calculated from NHANES 2002 data. US Department of Health and Human Services.

[2] Stengle J. Report of the American Heart Association. December 30, 2004.

[3] Buchwald H, Avidor Y, Braunwald E, et al. Bariatric surgery: a systematic review and meta-analysis. JAMA 2004;292:1724–37.

[4] Straker D. What is quality? Available at: http://www.iqa.org/publication/c4-1-46.shtml. Accessed November, 2004.

[5] Brown T. Sting ray success. Available at: http://www.iqa.org/publication/c4-1-103.shtml. Accessed November, 2004.

[6] Society of Interventional Radiology Standards of Practice Committee. Guidelines for establishing a quality assurance program in vascular and interventional radiology. J Vasc Interv Radiol 2003;14:S203–7.

[7] Agency for Healthcare Research and Quality. Clinical practice guidelines archive. Available at: http://www.ahrq.gov/clinic/cpgarchv.htm.

[8] Steinbrook MD. Surgry for severe obesity. N Engl J Med 2004;350:1075–9.

[9] Stockbridge P. Making medicine with quality assurance. Available at: http://www.iqa.org/publication/c4-1-43.shtml. Accessed November, 2004.

[10] Quality assurance manager in close-up. Available at: http://www.prospects.ac.uk/cms. Accessed November, 2004.

ELSEVIER
SAUNDERS

SURGICAL
CLINICS OF
NORTH AMERICA

Surg Clin N Am 85 (2005) 773–787

Laparoscopic Adjustable Gastric Banding: Evolving Clinical Experience

Eric J. DeMaria, MD*, Mohammad K. Jamal, MD

Division of General Surgery, Department of Surgery,
Center for Minimally Invasive Surgery and the Obesity Surgery Program,
Virginia Commonwealth University/Medical College of Virginia,
Box 980428, Richmond, VA 23298, USA

Laparoscopic surgical techniques have dramatically evolved over the last two decades and have created a worldwide revolution in the field of bariatric surgery (see Appendix). Although laparoscopic techniques have progressively replaced the open approach to bariatric surgery, great disparity exists regarding the preferred procedure around the world. The gastric bypass [1–3] and duodenal switch [4] currently represent nearly 80% to 90% of laparoscopic bariatric procedures in the United States and Canada [5], whereas laparoscopic gastric restrictive procedures still represent the majority of bariatric procedures performed in Europe [6–7]. Several reasons may explain this disparity: most important of all, different dietary habits in European patients may explain the potential for a better response to gastric restrictive procedures. Secondly, the majority of European patients presenting for weight loss surgery have a body mass index (BMI) between 35 and 50 kg/m^2, with only a small minority of patients being super-obese (BMI > 50 kg/m^2). This is in contrast to the United States population, in which a higher BMI among patients is more common. Gastric restriction typically fails in these super-obese patients, and malabsorptive bariatric procedures remain the mainstay of surgical treatment in this group [8–9].

Laparoscopic adjustable gastric banding (LAGB) was first introduced in the early 1990s as a potentially safe, controllable, and reversible method for achieving significant weight loss in the severely obese. The Lap-Band system (INAMED Health, formerly BioEnterics Corporation, Santa Barbara, California) is the device most commonly used. After 10 years of experience with LAGB in treating more than 100,000 patients around

---

* Corresponding author.
E-mail address: edemaria@hsc.vcu.edu (E.J. DeMaria).

0039-6109/05/$ - see front matter © 2005 Elsevier Inc. All rights reserved.
doi:10.1016/j.suc.2005.04.008   *surgical.theclinics.com*

the world it is timely to review the existing data on this procedure derived from European, Australian, and American studies and compare their results. Special emphasis is placed on clinical outcomes and reported complications of LAGB. In general, international studies support use of the LAGB procedure, while American studies are generally better designed but more equivocal in their results.

European studies

One of the biggest European LAGB experiences comes from Italy. Angrisani and colleagues [10] reported their experience with 1265 patients undergoing LAGB. These included 258 male and 1007 female patients with a mean BMI of 44.1 kg/m². Follow-up was obtained at 6, 12, 18, 24, 36, and 48 months, and mean BMI was 38.4, 35.1, 33.1, 30.2, 32.1, and 31.5 kg/m², respectively; hence the mean reduction in BMI over 4 years was 12.6 kg/m². The percentage of patients observed at each follow-up was greater than 60%. There was no intraoperative or complication-related mortality. Postoperative mortality was 0.55% (n = 7) for causes not specifically related to LAGB implantation. The open conversion rate was 1.7% (n = 22). LAGB-related complications occurred in 11.3% (n = 143) with pouch dilatation diagnosed in 65 patients (5.2%), band erosion in 24 patients (1.9%), and port or connecting tube-port complications in 54 patients (4.2%). Several of these complications required reoperation or revision.

Weiner and colleagues [11] reported the German experience with LAGB in 984 consecutive patients over an 8-year period. In this series, initial body weight was 132 kg and BMI was 46.8 kg/m². Retro-gastric placement was performed in the initial 577 patients after which the pars flaccida or peri-gastric technique was used in the remaining 407 patients. Median follow-up was 55 months, and there were no conversions or mortalities. Mean excess weight loss (EWL) was 59.3% after 8 years with a drop in BMI from 46.8 to 32.3 kg/m² in this group. Five of the first 100 patients to receive LAGB underwent band removal with 3/5 patients converted to laparoscopic Roux-en-Y gastric bypass (LRYGBP) with successful weight loss after the re-do surgery. Fourteen patients were switched to a "banded" LRYGBP for failed weight loss. The quality of life indices were improved in nearly 82% of the first 100 patients. The best results were achieved during the first 2 years after LAGB. Early complications reported in this series were gastric perforation (n = 1) and slippage (n = 1); late complications included slippage requiring reinterventions (n = 17) during the following years.

Similar results have been reported by several others [12–15]. In a series of 1250 patients, O'Brien and Dixon [12] reported Lap-Band placement to be a very safe procedure with a mortality rate of 1 in 2000, only 10% of the published mortality rate of gastric bypass. Although the early complication rate was very low, late complications of prolapse or erosions were frequent, particularly during their early experience. Weight loss was maximal during the first 2 to 3 years after surgery and averaged 56% of EWL at 5 years. This was in comparison to the RYGB where EWL was reported to be 59% at 5 years. Major improvements in comorbid conditions were reported in association with weight loss after Lap-Band placement in these series; this was particularly true for resolution of type 2 diabetes with improvement in insulin resistance and pancreatic beta-cell function. Gastroesophageal reflux disease, obstructive sleep apnea, and depression were other major comorbid conditions that showed marked improvement. Another review by Favretti and colleagues [13] showed similar results in a series of 830 patients. The initial mean body weight in this group was 127 kg with a BMI of 46 kg/m^2. The reported conversion rate was 2.7% without a mortality with major complications requiring reoperation developing in 3.9% (n = 36). These included early complications with 1 gastric perforation (requiring band removal) and 1 gastric slippage (requiring repositioning). Late complications included 17 gastric slippages (treated by band repositioning in 12 and band removal in 5), 9 malpositionings (all treated by band repositioning), 4 gastric erosions (all treated by band removal), 3 psychologic intolerance (requiring band removal), and 1 HIV sero-conversion (band removed). A minor complication requiring reoperation in 91 patients (11%) was reservoir leakage. On the negative side was a high incidence of failure, whereas an error in the manuscript suggested 20% of patients failed to lose at least 30% of excess weight, the actual calculation from the authors' table of 3-year results revealed this failure incidence to be nearly 30%. The authors suggest failure arose in most cases from patients losing "compliance with dietetic, psychological and surgical advice"—which, of course, represents an opinion rather than something proven by their analysis. It should be remembered that recidivism is a well-known characteristic of clinically severe obesity and, while surgeons often blame their patients for their failures, the ideal bariatric procedure would perform independently of patient compliance to minimize poor long-term weight loss outcomes. The overall reduction in BMI in this study was significant—from the initial 46.4 to 37.3 at 1 year, 36.4 at 2 years, 36.8 at 3 years and 36.4 kg/m^2 at 5 years. Clearly some patients did well in the 5-year term, while many did not.

In the series of 400 patients undergoing LAGB reported by Chevallier and colleagues [14], mean BMI fell from 43.8 to 32.7 kg/m^2 with a mean EWL of 52.7% at 2 years follow-up. Mean operative time was 116 minutes, mean hospital stay was 4.55 days, and there were no mortalities. There were 12 conversions (3%) with complications requiring an abdominal reoperation in 10% of the patients. These included gastric perforation (n = 2), gastric necrosis (n = 1), slippage (n = 31), incisional hernia (n = 2), and reconnection of the tube (n = 4).

Only a few authors have reported data on resolution of major comorbidities after Lap Band placement. In a series of 295 patients with a mean BMI of 45 kg/m^2 undergoing the LAGB, reduction in comorbidity was scaled relative to the preoperative comorbidity level as having been cured, improved, unchanged, or worsened [16]. The preoperative frequencies of comorbidities in this study were typical of most obesity surgery series and included hypertension (52%), diabetes (20%), dyspnea (85%), peripheral edema (63%), sleep apnea (36%), arthralgia (89%), gastroesophageal reflux (57%), reduced self-esteem (95%), reduced general physical performance (96%), hyperlipidemia (39%), hyperuricemia (36%), and menstrual problems (22%). Excess weight loss was 40% after 1 year, 46% after 2 years, 47% after 3 years, and 54% after 4 years follow-up. After 4 years, the rates of cure/improvement of the comorbidities were: hypertension 58%/42%, diabetes 75%/8%, dyspnea 85%/12%, arthralgia 52%/24%, reflux 79%/11%, self-esteem 45%/39% and general physical performance 58%/33%. Significant improvement was also found in stress incontinence, sleep apnea, peripheral edema, and regulation of menstruation. Greater weight loss was associated with a greater reduction in dyspnea and arthralgia, improved self-esteem, and physical performance, whereas hypertension, diabetes, reflux, and edema improved independently of the amount of weight loss. In essence, major comorbidities were cured in 50% to 80% and improved in 10% to 40% of all patients undergoing the LAGB in this series.

Another device, the so-called "Swedish adjustable gastric band" (SAGB, Ehicon Endo-Surgery, Cincinatti, Ohio, USA), has been compared with other laparoscopic bariatric procedures, including the gastric bypass, LAGB, and vertical band gastroplasty [15]. In a series of 454 patients undergoing laparoscopic SAGB, the average weight loss was 35.5 kg after 1 year, reaching an average of 54 kg after 3 years. Mean EWL was 72% after 3 years, and the BMI decreased from 46.7 to 28.1 kg/m^2. Marked improvement in comorbidities was also reported in patients undergoing the SAGB. Complications requiring reoperation occurred in 7.9%, whereas there were no mortalities. In a series of 824 patients undergoing laparoscopic SAGB over a 5-year period, preoperative data, postoperative weight loss, and long-term complications were prospectively obtained for analysis [17]. The mean preoperative BMI of these patients was 43 kg/m^2. Excess weight loss of >50% was achieved in 82.9% of the patients after initial treatment. At the end of the follow-up period, mean EWL was 30%, 41%, 49%, 55%, and 57% after 1, 2, 3, 4, and 5 years, respectively. There were no intra- or postoperative deaths reported in the series. The intraoperative conversion rate was 5.2%, whereas the perioperative complication rate was 1.2%. Long-term complications occurred in 191 patients (23.2%), related primarily to the band (16.4%) or to the access port or tubing (6.8%).

Although the lower degree of weight loss following LAGB has discouraged use of the device in super-obese patients, some encouraging results have been reported in this population. Angrisani and colleagues [18] reported their retrospective analysis of the multicenter Italian experience with the LAGB performed in patients with a BMI above 50 kg/m^2. In this group of 239 patients with a mean age of 37 years and a mean BMI of 54.6 kg/m^2 undergoing the LAGB, follow-up was obtained at 6, 12, 24, 36, and 48 months; at these time periods, mean BMI was 46.7, 43.9, 42.2, 41.9, and 39.3 kg/m^2, respectively. At the same intervals, the mean EWL was 24.1, 34.1, 38.8, 38.9, and 52.9%, respectively. The conversion rate was 5.4%, whereas postoperative complications occurred in 9.0% of patients. Serious comorbidities had completely resolved in 60% of the patients at the end of 1-year follow-up. Interestingly, the number of patients with less than 25% EWL at 12, 24, 36, and 48 months follow-up were 34, 10, 4, and 0, respectively. Based on these results, it appears that even though super-obese patients undergoing the LAGB remain morbidly obese (BMI > 35 kg/m^2) at the end of the 4-year follow-up, in the short term most patients lose their comorbidities with a low morbidity and mortality rate.

Positive outcomes in superobese patients have led some to suggest that LAGB should be the preferred initial procedure for all morbidly obese patients, with more complex gastrointestinal procedures reserved for weight loss failures only. In fact, many bariatric surgeons in the United States today are allowing patients to choose their own surgical procedure. This provides insight into the relative lack of clear data demonstrating how to successfully tailor the choice of operation to the individual patient in this rapidly growing new specialty. A flaw in this line of thinking also rests in the assessment of surgical risk for revisional versus primary procedures. Revision to proximal gastric bypass from a failed primary gastroplasty procedure carries a higher risk of complications, particularly anastomotic leak, than does a primary gastric bypass operation. A similar increase in the risk of postoperative complications has been demonstrated after failed LAGB [19]. Finally, one could question the logic of performing a procedure on all candidates that has been shown to carry a 20% to 30% failure rate [13] when it would make more sense to analyze subgroups of morbidly obese patients to determine predictors that would signal that successful long-term weight loss is more likely.

Proponents of LAGB claim that it is a technically less challenging surgical procedure than the gastric bypass and that most re-operations for complications can be performed laparoscopically with low morbidity and short hospitalizations. Szold and Abu-Abeid [20] reported preliminary results of their experience with LAGB in 715 patients followed up prospectively for management of perioperative and long-term complications. The mean age of the patients was 34 years, with a mean BMI of 43.1 kg/m^2. Their mean operative time was 78 minutes, with a postoperative hospitalization time of 1.2 days. There were six intraoperative complications (0.8%), eight early postoperative complications (1.1%), and no deaths. Late complications included band slippage or pouch dilation in 53 patients (7.4%), band erosion in 3 patients, and port complications in 18 patients. In 57 patients (7.9%), 69 major reoperations were performed. Six patients (0.84%) underwent reoperation during the first 3 postoperative days: one for a bleeding trocar site, and five for band repositioning because of band malposition and outlet obstruction. All early repositioning procedures were performed through a laparotomy. Band dislodgment or pouch dilation occurred in 53 patients (7.4%). All these patients had radiographic studies to prove band dislodgment, and all underwent laparoscopic surgery for band repositioning or band removal. The reasons for band removal were patient request or patient refusal of regular follow-up evaluation in 20 patients, band erosion in 3 patients and previous band repositioning in 9 patients. In addition, 18 procedures were performed on the ports, most with the patient under local anesthesia. The data for 181 patients with a follow-up period longer than 2 years were studied to obtain long-term follow-up information. A total of 121 patients (66.8%) were available for a mean follow-up period of 30 months with a drop in BMI from 43.3 to 32.1 kg/m^2.

United States experience

LAGB is the most commonly performed bariatric procedure in Europe and Australia and has been shown to result in significant long-term weight loss and resolution of comorbidities. However, clinical trials sponsored by the US Food and Drug Administration (FDA) with the Lap-Band system did not reproduce the results of studies performed elsewhere in the world.

The first FDA-monitored clinical trial to evaluate the Lap-Band system in morbidly obese patients began in April 1995 and was called the Trial-A (or Lap-Band Adjustable Gastric Banding System for Treatment of Clinically Severe Obesity). This trial included eight centers and 299 patients who were followed for 36 months. Of the 299 patients, 292 received the Lap-Band whereas 7 received an earlier version of the device called the adjustable silicone gastric band (ASGB). Of the 292 Lap-Band patients in Trial-A, 89% (n = 259) had the band placed laparoscopically using the peri-gastric technique whereas 11% (n = 33) had the band implanted by way of laparotomy. The average % EWL in Trial-A was 26.5 at 6 months, 34.5 at 12 months, 37.8 at 24 months and 36.2 at 36 months.

We reported our clinical experience with the Lap-Band at one of the eight original United States centers performing LAGB as part of the FDA-monitored Trial-A [21]. Thirty-seven patients were enrolled and underwent laparoscopic placement of the Lap-Band with successful placement in 36 patients. One patient required an open conversion to a gastric bypass following an intraoperative gastric perforation. Patients were followed up for up to 4 years after surgery for weight loss and resolution of comorbidities. Five patients (14%) had a mean follow-up of

2 years but at last available follow-up had achieved only 18% EWL. The LAGB devices were removed in 15 (41%) patients 10 days to 42 months after surgery. Four of these patients underwent simple removal, whereas 11 were converted to a gastric bypass. The most common reason for removal was inadequate weight loss in the presence of a functioning band. The primary reasons for removal in others were infection, leakage from the inflatable silicone ring causing inadequate weight loss and band slippage. Bands were also removed in two others as a result of symptoms related to esophageal dilatation. Significant esophageal dilatation developed in 18 of 25 patients (71%) who underwent preoperative and long-term postoperative contrast evaluation. Of these, 13 (72%) patients had prominent dysphagia, vomiting or reflux symptoms. Of the remaining 21 patients with bands, 8 desired band removal and conversion to a gastric bypass for inadequate weight loss. Six of the remaining patients had persistent morbid obesity 2 years after surgery but refused to undergo further surgery. Overall, only 4 patients achieved a BMI of less than 35 or at least a 50% reduction in excess weight. Thus the overall need for band removal and conversion to gastric bypass in this series exceeded 50%. Based on these results, the Lap-Band was not felt to be an effective and durable surgical modality for the treatment of morbid obesity. Inadequate weight loss was more prominent in the African American cohort for reasons unknown but was consistent with the general observation that this population demonstrates inferior weight loss after other forms of obesity surgery as well.

Regarding conversion of LAGB to gastric bypass [19], the conversions were technically difficult to perform and fraught with serious complications. Three patients developed intraoperative gastro-jejunal leaks identified during endoscopy and requiring intraoperative repair, and another patient developed postoperative bleeding requiring re-exploration. One patient that was converted laparoscopically developed a gastro-jejunal anastomotic leak postoperatively that healed with 3 weeks of outpatient total parenteral nutrition. Three of 5 patients requiring open conversion developed ventral hernias necessitating repair. Of the 18 patients in our series who remain under treatment with the Lap-Band, the mean percentage of EWL is only 32% and most of these patients no longer will return to the medical center for follow-up. Hence, this early experience with the Lap-Band system was associated with a high frequency of inadequate weight loss and resolution of comorbidities. Conversion to gastric bypass in this subset of patients was found to be technically challenging but resulted in superior weight loss in a shorter time period.

The second FDA-monitored clinical trial, called Trial-B (Clinical Evaluation of the Lap-Band System in Clinically Severe Obese Patients) began in 1999 and also followed patients for up to 36 months [22]. The single published report from Trial-B involved 63 patients who underwent LAGB between March 1999 and June 2001. All of these patients underwent laparoscopic placement of the Lap-Band with placement done by way of the classic high peri-gastric dissection above the lesser sac. Operative time decreased from a mean of 197 minutes for the first 10 patients to 120 minutes for the last group, with an average hospital stay of 1.4 days. The average % EWL in the Trial-B patients was 27.2 at 6 months, 38.3 at 12 months, 46.6 at 24 months, and 53.6 at 36 months. Before surgery, 46 of 63 patients (73%) suffered from serious comorbidity. Following LAGB, all categories showed marked improvement.

More complications occurred in Trial-A compared with the published 63 patients in trial-B. When compared with Trial-B, nausea or vomiting occurred in 51% of patients in trial A compared with 23%; gastroesophageal reflux occurred in 34% versus 2%; gastric prolapse (band slippage)/pouch dilatation occurred in 24% versus 5%; stoma obstruction occurred in 14% versus 0%; esophageal dilatation occurred in 10% versus 6%; port problems occurred in 15% versus 8%; and erosions occurred in 1% in both groups. Perioperative complications in Trial-B included one intraoperative gastric perforation that was closed and did not prevent band placement. Two deaths occurred during the course of Trial-A: one due to "mixed drug intoxication" a week after explantation and the other to multiple pulmonary emboli a day after explantation of the Lap-Band and conversion to a RYGBP. No deaths were reported among the 63 Trial-B patients.

Doherty and colleagues [23] reported their experience with both the ASGB and the Lap-Band in a prospective study of 62 patients over an 8-year period. Some of their Lap-Band patients also entered the FDA-monitored Trial-A. Forty ASGB and 22 Lap-Bands were implanted in this group of patients with a mean weight of 145 kg and a mean BMI of 49 kg/m². In the ASGB cohort, the BMI decreased from 50 to 36 kg/m² over a 3-year period and then increased to 44 kg/m² at 8 years after operation. In the Lap-Band cohort, the BMI decreased from 47 to 40 kg/m² at 1 year and then increased to 43 kg/m² at 6 years after operation. There were no operative mortalities. Thirty intra-abdominal re-operations were necessary to correct complications related to the implanted ASGB or Lap-Band. The adverse events included infected band (1.6%), obstructive aneurysmal deformity of the inflatable bladder component of the band (3.2%, n = 2 ASGB), enlarged pouch with obstructive angulation of the outlet channel (17.7%, n = 11; 7 ASGB, 4 Lap-Bands), herniation of the distal stomach through the band into the posterior lesser sac causing obstruction (22.6%, n = 14; 11 ASGB, 3 Lap-Band). Seven subjects voluntarily withdrew from the study because of minimal or no weight loss. Twenty-seven implantable devices (18 ASGB, 9 Lap-Band) were removed by the time of publication. After 116 months, only 26 subjects (42% of participants) remained. Their conclusions suggested that the ASGB or the Lap-Band device were not effective or durable modalities for the surgical treatment of morbid obesity.

An initial clinical series reported by Ren and colleagues [24] provided short-term data on nearly 500 patients undergoing the LAGB at 4 US medical centers. Of these, 115 patients were followed for at least 9 months and 43 for at least 12 months. The reported % EWL was 35.6 at 9 months and 41.6 at 12 months. The average BMI decreased from 47.5 kg/m^2 to 38.8 kg/m^2 in 9 months and from 47.5 kg/m^2 to 37.3 kg/m^2 in 12 months. There were no deaths related to the insertion of the device. Conversion to an open procedure was necessary in 1 patient (1%). Acute perioperative complications occurred in 4 patients (3%) and included 2 stoma obstructions, 1 hemorrhage, and a case of pneumonia. The acute stoma obstructions, secondary to edema, were treated conservatively with intravenous hydration and resolved spontaneously. Wound infection occurred in 5 patients (4%). These were conservatively managed with oral antibiotics and resolved in all but one patient in whom a port abscess developed that required port removal 3 weeks postoperatively and subsequent port replacement 6 months postoperatively. There were no device-related mortalities in the group, but 12 patients developed complications requiring operative management (13%). These included eight port displacements or tubing breaks (7%), two elective explantations (2%), two gastric prolapse (2%) and a gastric pouch dilatation (1%).

Another series by Ren and colleagues described favorable early results of LAGB at two American academic centers [25]. In this series of 445 patients, the mean BMI was 49.6 kg/m^2, with a mean total body weight of 299 lbs. One case required conversion to a laparotomy for bleeding, whereas the rest were completed laparoscopically. Mean length of stay was 1.1 days and there was one death. Additional complications in this series included band slippage in 14 patients (3.1%), gastric obstruction without slip in 12 (2.7%), port migration in 2 (0.4%), tubing disconnections in 3 (0.7%), and port infection in 5 (1.1%). Two bands (0.4%) were removed because of intra-abdominal abscess 2 months after placement. There was one band erosion (0.2%) and no clinically significant esophageal dilation. Ninety-nine patients have 1-year follow-up and have lost an average of 44.3% excess body weight. Although no data was provided on resolution of comorbidities, this series suggested comparable weight loss to most European studies.

A comparative study of LAGB with RYGBP was reported by Biertho and colleagues [26]. In this analysis, 456 patients undergoing the LRYGBP at a United States center were compared with 805 LAGB performed in European institutions [23]. Body mass index, complication rates, mortality, and excess weight loss after 3, 6, 12, and 18 months were obtained. The 805 patients selected for this study underwent laparoscopic SAGB (Obtech, Ethicon Endo-Surgery, Cincinatti, Ohio, USA) performed as the initial surgical treatment of their obesity. Patients with a BMI above 50 kg/m^2 were usually considered for an open gastric bypass. Preoperative BMI was 49.4 kg/m^2 in the RYGBP group and 42.2 kg/m^2 in the LAGB group; the perioperative major complication rates were 2.0% versus 1.3%, and the early postoperative major complication rates were 4.2% versus 1.7%. Mortality rate was 0.4% in the RYGBP group versus 0% in the LAGB group. The global EWL was 36.3% for RYGBP versus 14.7% for LAGB at 3 months, 51.6% versus 21.9% at 6 months, 67.0% versus 33.3% at 12 months and 74.6% versus 40.4% at 18 months, respectively. Long-term follow-up for the LAGB group showed an EWL of 47% at 2 years, 56% at 3 years and 58% at 4 years. The EWL at 3, 6, 12 and 18 months was statistically superior in the LGB group, for all BMI ranges studied.

Summary

Surgical procedures for the treatment of morbid obesity fall into one of two categories: bypass and restrictive procedures (or a combination of both). The restrictive procedures usually are simple, technically easier operations with low complication rates, but the suggestion has been made that they ultimately fail to be effective in the long term [27]. The procedures require banding of the gastric outlet via placement of a foreign body such as a silastic ring, an adjustable silicone band or prosthetic mesh and generally require some patient cooperation to maintain a restricted diet and avoid forced overfeeding and frequent vomiting, which tend to enlarge the proximal stomach or damage the restrictive device, rendering the procedure nonfunctional. Restrictive procedures are only effective in reducing the volume of solid food consumed by the patient. Liquid and semisolid, high-calorie foods can often pass through the banded outlet without creating a sense of satiety. This enables some patients to maintain or re-gain the excessive weight, making these procedures ineffective, particularly for the treatment of morbidly obese sweet-eaters.

In contrast, bypass procedures are aimed essentially at altering absorption to create a "controlled" state of malabsorption. Several procedures, including biliopancreatic diversion with or without duodenal switch, produce some degree of malabsorption by reducing the contact of digested food with the small bowel, pancreatic and biliary secretions, or both. These procedures theoretically enable the patient to continue eating an unrestricted diet and still lose weight. These procedures are generally major undertakings and require the formation of fundamental changes in the structure of the gastrointestinal tract. Furthermore, the degree of malabsorption is difficult to predict, and in some patients, the result is an undesirable degree of malabsorption necessitating reoperations and modifications to the original procedure.

Gastric bypass has elements of both restriction and malabsorption; however, given our evolving knowledge of gut adaptation, one would be hard-pressed to prove that the degree of intestinal bypass involved (100–200 cm) provides significant nutrient malabsorption in the long term. Gastric bypass does create malabsorption of important micronutrients, including calcium, iron and vitamin B_{12}, which must be supplemented in the patient's diet. In addition, the altered anatomy reliably produces altered gut absorption leading to symptoms of dumping syndrome in response to high-calorie sweets intake. This likely remains an important difference from pure gastric restriction and explains some of the greater weight loss that accompanies the gastric bypass and makes it the gold standard procedure for treatment of obesity.

The real appeal of LAGB is in its ease of performance from a technical standpoint, making it an achievable laparoscopic treatment option even for high-risk patients. Similarly, the lack of any intestinal anastomosis removes one catastrophic complication from the long list of potential risks to the morbidly obese patient undergoing surgery. Overall, the world literature suggests the LAGB is a beneficial operation with an acceptable complication rate. It is certainly superior to other forms of nonoperative treatment that uniformly fail to correct morbid obesity. Data are emerging to clarify the long-term potential for weight loss, which has been reported to be around 50% of excess. It appears likely that some technical complications such as stomach slippage have been minimized by improved surgical techniques.

The critical factor in long-term success after LAGB is likely to be assiduous multidisciplinary follow-up. Band adjustment strategies have evolved with increasing experience in the United States and around the world, and these appear critical to weight loss success, as is patient compliance with dietary restrictions and physical activity. Unfortunately, little clinical research has focused on the critical component of band adjustment. No long-term data exist to determine the potential for complications of the device in the US, including risks of band erosion and esophageal dilatation [21]. Furthermore, the disappointing history of the vertical-banded gastroplasty procedure in the United States, a similar restrictive operation for obesity, in which weight loss failure and weight re-gain became common outcomes [27], sends a warning that long-term data must be collected and analyzed to confirm the durability of the lap band device. Short-term clinical experience with the Lap-Band system in this country does suggest the device is a safe and potentially—although not conclusively—effective treatment for morbid obesity with results beginning to parallel those seen in other countries. The lap band procedure may not be the best surgical option in certain patient subgroups, including super-obese patients, diabetics (who have a higher cure rate and greater weight loss with gastric bypass), patients with hiatal hernia or significant gastroesophageal reflux disease and African American patients [21]. The combination of proper surgical technique and close patient follow-up with frequent band adjustments performed in a comprehensive bariatric program setting may make this device an effective surgical treatment of morbid obesity.

Appendix

European experience with the Lap-Band/SAGB

Study	No. of patients	Mean age (years)	Mean preoperative BMI (kg/m²)	Mean duration of follow-up (months)	Mean postoperative BMI (kg/m²)	% EWL	Conversion rate (%)	Mortality (%)
Angrisani et al [10]	1265	38	44.1	48	31.5	N/I	1.7	0.55
Weiner et al [11]	984	37	46.8	55	32.3	59	0	0
Favretti et al [13]	830	37	46	60	36.4	N/I	2.7	0
Chevallier et al [14]	400	40	43.8	24	32.7	52.7	3	0
Frigg et al [16]	295	41	45	44	N/I	54	N/I	N/I
Angrisani et al [18]	239	37	54.6	48	39.3	52.9	5.4	N/I
Szold and Abu-Abeid [20]	715	34	43.1	24	32.1	N/I	N/I	0
Martikainen et al [28]	123	44	49	55	N/I	N/I	N/I	N/I
Mittermair et al [15][a]	454	NA	46.7	30	28.1	72	N/I	0

Abbreviation: N/I, not identified on review.
[a] SAGB only.

Lap-Band complications in European studies

Study	Pouch dilatation (%)	Band erosion (%)	Band migration (%)	Slippage (%)	Esophageal dilatation (%)	Gastric perforation (%)	Gastric necrosis (%)	Port/tube problems (%)	Pulmonary embolism (%)
Angrisani et al [18]	5.2	1.9	N/I	N/I	N/I	N/I	N/I	4.2	N/I
Weiner et al [11]	N/I	N/I	N/I	3.7	N/I	0.1	N/I	N/I	N/I
Favretti et al [13]	N/I	0.5	1.1	2.2	N/I	0.1	N/I	11	N/I
Chevallier et al [29]	N/I	N/I	N/I	7.8	N/I	0.5	0.25	0.09	N/I
Szold and Abu-Abeid [20]	7.4	0.4	N/I	N/I	N/I	N/I	N/I	2.5	N/I
Chevallier et al [14]	N/I	N/I	0.3	7.8	0.2	0.4	0.1	2.1	0.2

Abbreviation: N/I, not identified on review.

US experience with the Lap-Band

Study	No. of patients	Mean age (years)	Mean preoperative BMI (kg/m²)	Mean duration of follow-up (months)	Mean postoperative BMI (kg/m²)	% EWL	Conversion rate (%)	Mortality (%)
DeMaria et al [21]	37	38	44.5	36	34	44	2.7	0
Doherty et al [23]	22	34	47	72	43	15	N/I	0
Ren et al [24]	445	42	52.7	12	39.3	44.3	0.2	0.2
FDA Trial-A	292	38	47.4	36	38.7	36.2	11	0.7
FDA Trial-B	63	40	48.8	36	N/I	53.6	0	0

Abbreviation: N/I, not identified on review.

Lap-Band complications in United States studies

Study	Nausea/ Vomiting (%)	Reflux (%)	Pouch dilatation (%)	Band erosion (%)	Band migration (%)	Slippage (%)	Esophageal dilatation (%)	Gastric perforation (%)	Gastric necrosis (%)	Port/tube problems (%)	Pulmonary embolism (%)
DeMaria et al [21]	N/I	N/I	N/I	N/I	N/I	(8.1)	(67.6)	(2.7)	N/I	(0.11)	N/I
Doherty et al [23]	N/I	N/I	(18.2)	N/I	(13.6)	N/I	N/I	N/I	N/I	N/I	N/I
Ren et al [24]	N/I	N/I	N/I	0.2	N/I	3.1	N/I	N/I	N/I	2.3	N/I
FDA Trial-A	51	34	24	1	N/I	N/I	10	N/I	N/I	15	1
FDA Trial-B	23	2	5	1	N/I	14.2	6	1.5	N/I	8	0

Abbreviation: N/I, not identified on review.

References

[1] Wittgrove AC, Clark GW, Tremblay LJ. Laparoscopic gastric bypass, Roux-en-Y: preliminary report of five cases. Obes Surg 1994;4:353–7.

[2] Wittgrove AC, Clark GW. Laparoscopic gastric bypass Roux en Y in 500 patients: technique and results, with 3–60 months follow-up. Obes Surg 2000;10:233–9.

[3] Schauer PR, Ikramuddin S, Gourash W, et al. Outcomes after laparoscopic Roux-en-Y gastric bypass for morbid obesity. Ann Surg 2000;232:515–29.

[4] Ren CJ, Patterson E, Gagner M. Early results of laparoscopic biliopancreatic diversion with duodenal switch: a case series of 40 consecutive patients. Obes Surg 2000;10:514–23.

[5] Schauer PR, Ikramuddin S. Laparoscopic surgery for morbid obesity. Surg Clin North Am 2001;81:1145–79.

[6] Leffler E, Gustavsson S, Karlson BM. Time trends in obesity surgery 1987 through 1996 in Sweden: a population-based study. Obes Surg 2000;10:543–8.

[7] Toppino M, Mistrangelo M, Bonansone V, et al. Obesity surgery: 4-years results from the Italian Registry (R.I.C.O.). Obes Surg 2000;10:320.

[8] Capella JF, Capella RF. The weight reduction operation of choice: vertical banded gastroplasty or gastric bypass? Am J Surg 1996;171:74–9.

[9] Fox SR, Oh KH, Fox KS. Vertical banded gastroplasty and distal gastric bypass as primary procedures: a comparison. Obes Surg 1996;6:421–5.

[10] Angrisani L, Alkilani M, Basso N. Laparoscopic Italian experience with the Lap-Band. Obes Surg 2001;11:307–10.

[11] Weiner R, Blanco-Engert R, Weiner S. Outcome after laparoscopic adjustable gastric banding—8 years experience. Obes Surg 2003;13:427–34.

[12] O'Brien PE, Dixon JB. Lap-band: outcomes and results. J Laparoendosc Adv Surg Tech A 2003;13:265–70.

[13] Favretti F, Cadiere GB, Segato G. Laparoscopic banding: selection and technique in 830 patients. Obes Surg 2002;12:385–90.

[14] Chevallier JM, Zinzindohoue F, Elian N. Adjustable gastric banding in a public university hospital: prospective analysis of 400 patients. Obes Surg 2002;12:93–9.

[15] Mittermair RP, Weiss H, Nehoda H. Laparoscopic Swedish adjustable gastric banding: 6-year follow-up and comparison to other laparoscopic bariatric procedures. Obes Surg 2003;13:412–7.

[16] Frigg A, Peterli R, Peters T. Reduction in co-morbidities 4 years after laparoscopic adjustable gastric banding. Obes Surg 2004;14:216–23.

[17] Steffen R, Biertho L, Ricklin T. Laparoscopic Swedish adjustable gastric banding: a five-year prospective study. Obes Surg 2003;13:404–11.

[18] Angrisani L, Furbetta F, Doldi SB. Results of the Italian multicenter study on 239 super-obese patients treated by adjustable gastric banding. Obes Surg 2002;12:846–50.

[19] Kothari SN, DeMaria EJ, Sugerman HJ, et al. Lap-band failures: conversion to gastric bypass and their preliminary outcomes. Surgery 2002;131:625–9.

[20] Szold A, Abu-Abeid S. Laparoscopic adjustable silicone gastric banding for morbid obesity: results and complications in 715 patients. Surg Endosc 2002;16:230–3.

[21] DeMaria EJ, Sugerman HJ, Meador JG, et al. High failure rate after laparoscopic adjustable silicone gastric banding for treatment of morbid obesity. Ann Surg 2001;233:809–18.

[22] Rubenstein RB. Laparoscopic adjustable gastric banding at a US center with up to 3-year follow-up. Obes Surg 2002;12:380–4.

[23] Doherty C, Maher JW, Heitshusen DS. Long-term data indicate a progressive loss in efficacy of adjustable silicone gastric banding for the surgical treatment of morbid obesity. Surgery 2002;132:724–8.

[24] Ren CJ, Horgan S, Ponce J. US experience with the Lap-Band system. Am J Surg 2002;184: 46S–50S.

[25] Ren CJ, Weiner M, Allen JW. Favorable early results of gastric banding for morbid obesity: the American experience. Surg Endosc 2004;18:543–6.

[26] Biertho L, Steffen R, Ricklin T. Laparoscopic gastric bypass versus laparoscopic adjustable gastric banding: a comparative study of 1,200 cases. J Am Coll Surg 2003;197:536–47.

[27] Balsiger BM, Poggio JL, Mai J, et al. Ten and more years after vertical banded gastroplasty as primary operation for morbid obesity. J Gastrointest Surg 2000;4:598–605.

[28] Martikainen T, Pirinen E, Alhava E, Poikolainen E, et al. Long-term results, late complications and quality of life in a series of adjustable gastric banding. Obes Surg 2004 May;14(5):648–54.

[29] Chevallier JM, Zinzindohoue F, Douard R. Complications after laparoscopic adjustable gastric banding for morbid obesity: experience with 1,000 patients over 7 years. Obes Surg 2004 Mar;14(3):407–14.

ELSEVIER
SAUNDERS

SURGICAL
CLINICS OF
NORTH AMERICA

Surg Clin N Am 85 (2005) 789–805

Laparoscopic Adjustable Gastric Banding: An Attractive Option

David A. Provost, MD[a,b,*]

[a]Division of Gastrointestinal and Endocrine Surgery, Department of Surgery,
The University of Texas Southwestern Medical Center at Dallas,
5323 Harry Hines Boulevard, Dallas, TX 75039, USA
[b]Clinical Center for the Surgical Management of Obesity,
The University of Texas Southwestern Medical Center at Dallas,
5323 Harry Hines Boulevard, Dallas, TX 75039, USA

Obesity is a major health issue posing a difficult therapeutic challenge for clinicians in the United States. According to the Centers for Disease Control, more than two thirds of Americans are overweight, and nearly one third are obese [1]. Researchers and physicians are beginning to realize that obesity is a chronic condition, like hypertension or diabetes, influenced by genetic, metabolic, and environmental factors. The pathogenesis of morbid obesity involves more than just a lack of willpower or a sedentary lifestyle. Obesity contributes to the development of numerous life-threatening or disabling disorders including coronary heart disease, hypertension, type 2 diabetes mellitus, hyperlipidemia, degenerative joint disease, obstructive sleep apnea, and many types of cancer. Heavier men and women have an increased risk of death [2]. An estimated $45 billion is spent annually in the United States treating diseases associated with obesity, with total costs to society estimated at $140 billion. Annual health care costs are 44% higher for patients who have a body mass index (BMI) higher than 35 than in patients who have a BMI between 20 and 24. Significant weight reduction in the morbidly obese has been demonstrated to improve or reverse comorbid illness, while benefiting psychologic, social, and economic well-being.

The author has performed consultant work for INAMED Health and United States Surgical Corporation and received educational support from United States Surgical.

* Correspondence. Division of Gastrointestinal and Endocrine Surgery, Department of Surgery, the University of Texas Southwestern Medical Center at Dallas, 5323 Harry Hines Blvd. Dallas, TX 75039.

E-mail address: avid.provost@utsouthwestern.edu

doi:10.1016/j.suc.2005.04.004
surgical.theclinics.com

Tremendous resources are expended on diets and weight-reduction plans, with $30 billion annually spent on commercial weight-loss programs alone. Unfortunately, evidence demonstrating long-term success with medical, pharmacologic, diet, exercise, and behavioral therapies is absent. As a result, surgical procedures performed to treat morbid obesity have increased rapidly during the last decade, approaching 200,000 annually. Bariatric operations have been shown to produce sustained weight reduction with improvement or resolution in most obesity-related comorbidities [3], and two recent cohort trials have shown a survival benefit in patients undergoing Roux-en-Y gastric bypass (RYGB) [4,5]. In a population-based cohort study, Flum and colleagues [5] demonstrated a 33% reduction in mortality at 15 years in patients who had had a gastric bypass operation despite an operative mortality that approached 2%. An ideal weight loss operation would be one that could provide weight-loss benefits similar to the RYGB, improvements in comorbidities and survival, and reductions in perioperative morbidity and mortality. Laparoscopic adjustable gastric banding (LAGB) may prove to be that procedure.

History of gastric banding

The development of purely restrictive weight-loss operations evolved in an attempt to avoid the perioperative and long-term morbidity of the jejuno-ileal bypass and the early experience with gastric bypass. Initial attempts at gastric partitioning to create a gastric pouch, leading to a sensation of fullness with ingestion of small portions of food, were unsuccessful because of early weight regain. The introduction of the vertical banded gastroplasty (VBG) by Mason [6] in 1982 demonstrated that restrictive procedures could safely produce sustained weight reduction. Open gastric banding, initially using polypropylene or polyester mesh wrapped around the proximal stomach to create a restrictive pouch, achieved little support because of frequent outlet obstruction and band erosion. The simplicity of the procedure and the elimination of the reliance on staples to create the gastric partition were appealing. Use of an adjustable band first was reported in animal studies in 1982 [7], followed by the initial placement of an adjustable gastric band in a human by Kuzmak and colleagues [8] in 1986. Rapid advances in laparoscopic surgery in the early 1990s stimulated modifications of the Kuzmak band for laparoscopic placement, leading to the initial placement of the Lap-Band (INAMED Health, Santa Barbara, California) in a human by Belachew and colleagues [9] in September 1993. The Lap-Band System became available to trained surgeons internationally in 1994, and LAGB subsequently became the most frequently performed weight-loss operation in Europe, Australia, and Latin America. Food and Drug Administration (FDA) clinical trials were initiated in 1995, leading to FDA approval of the Lap-Band in the United States in June 2001.

LAGB provides the benefits of minimally invasive surgery for the surgical management of morbid obesity, with significantly lower perioperative morbidity and mortality than with RYGB or VBG [10]. Ease of insertion extends laparoscopic benefits to the extremes of obesity, with rapid recovery and potential reversibility.

Surgical technique of laparoscopic adjustable gastric band placement

The technique of LAGB placement has evolved from the initial descriptions by Belachew and colleagues [11] and Favretti and colleagues [12] as the result of attempts to minimize many of the late complications initially associated with the LAGB. The perigastric technique, as initially described, involved creating a window along the lesser curvature of the stomach 3 cm below the gastroesophageal junction (Fig. 1). This dissection was performed along the gastric wall medial to the neurovascular bundle of the lesser curvature. Attempts were made to maintain the dissection above the peritoneal reflection of the lesser omental bursa behind the stomach. The greater curvature dissection was performed superior to the first short gastric vessel. The dissection created a tunnel for band passage resulting in a 15- to 30-mL gastric pouch above the band. The greater curvature of the fundus was sutured over the band, typically with two sutures. The band stoma was then calibrated by injecting 1 to 2 mL saline into the inflatable balloon of the band, using a pressure gauge, the gastrostenometer, to determine proper pressure and position, to create a 12-mm stoma. With the perigastric technique, entry into or at the apex of the lesser omental sac posterior to the stomach creates a setting in which the posterior wall can slip through the band, creating a symptomatic prolapse [13], a complication reported in 23%

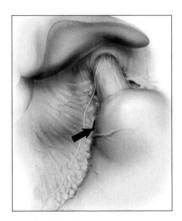 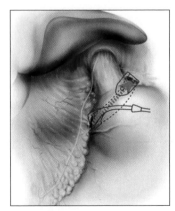

Fig. 1. Lap band perigastric 2. In the perigastric technique of lap band placement, the dissection is performed adjacent to the wall of the lesser curvature of the stomach, 3 cm below the gastroesophageal junction (*arrow*).

of patients in the FDA A Trial [14]. The problem of gastric prolapse was compounded by the partial inflation of the band at the time of surgery, increasing the likelihood of early vomiting with disruption of the fixation sutures. The larger pouch predisposed development of pouch dilation, and dissection close to the gastric wall along the lesser curvature often resulted in deserosalization, which may have led to the high incidence of band erosion observed with this technique.

In response to these complications, the method of LAGB placement has evolved into the pars flaccida technique (Fig. 2). Principles of the pars flaccida technique include the creation of a very small proximal pouch, posterior dissection just below the crura above the reflection of the bursa omentalis, improved anterior suture fixation of the fundus and anterior gastric wall over the band, and complete deflation of the band at the time of placement [15]. Candidates for LAGB must meet the indications for surgery as recommended by the National Institutes of Health Consensus Development Conference [16]. Intensive preoperative education regarding the risks and benefits of LAGB and dietary counseling are provided. The patient is placed on the operating table supine with adequate padding. The surgeon may operate from the patient's right side or from between the legs. Five or six ports are used, including a Nathanson liver retractor placed in the epigastrium. Dissection of the angle of His is performed well above the level of the short gastric vessels, freeing the gastrophrenic peritoneal attachments just lateral to the gastroesophageal junction to expose the left crus. This dissection is facilitated by excising the anterior fat pad overlying the gastroesophageal junction. The thin area of the gastrohepatic ligament, or pars flaccida, over the caudate lobe is divided, permitting identification of the base of the right crus. The peritoneum along the inferomedial border of the crus is incised, and a grasper is gently passed behind the gastroesoph-

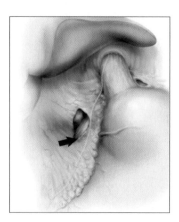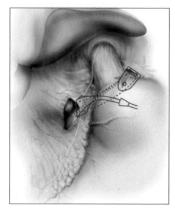

Fig. 2. Lap band pars flaccida 2. In the pars flaccida technique, posterior dissection is performed just below the right crux, above the peritoneal reflection of the bursa omentalis (*arrow*).

ageal junction to emerge behind the previously dissected angle of His. The band is inserted into the peritoneal cavity through a 15-mm trocar or, alternatively, may be passed through a 12-mm port site using the Ponce band passer. The end of the band is grasped by the grasper at the angle of His, and the tubing is pulled behind the gastroesophageal junction until the band encircles the proximal stomach. The tubing is passed through the band clasp, and the lock is seated. Gastrogastric sutures are placed to wrap the fundus and anterior gastric wall loosely over the band. At least three or four 2-0 sutures of braided polyester are placed from high on the fundus medially, stopping before the buckle of the band. Although the band is placed at the apex of the stomach, it is essential that the stomach, not the esophagus, be incorporated in the sutures superior to the band to achieve a sensation of satiety with meals. The end of the band tubing is brought out through a port site, the incision is lengthened, and a pocket is created subcutaneously on the anterior rectus sheath. The port is attached to the tubing, excess tubing is passed into the peritoneal cavity, and the port is secured to the anterior rectus sheath with permanent sutures. An upper gastrointestinal series is obtained postoperatively to document band position and to evaluate obstruction or gastroesophageal perforation. An overnight stay in the hospital is typical, although LAGB may be performed as an outpatient procedure.

Use of the pars flaccida technique has greatly decreased the incidence of gastric prolapse through the band, but incorporation of excessive perigastric fat within the band may result in postoperative outlet obstruction. This problem may be avoided by ensuring that the band rotates freely around the stomach before fixation and excising or incising the fat pad along the lesser curvature of the stomach [17]. Using the recently introduced Lap-Band VG System (INAMED Health, Santa Barbara, California), with a larger diameter, in patients who have large gastroesophageal fat pads may also minimize the incidence of postoperative obstruction.

Postoperative management of the laparoscopic adjustable gastric band

Although proper surgical technique is essential to minimize late complications of the LAGB, weight loss depends on postoperative follow-up and appropriate band adjustments. Frequent adjustments often are necessary to maintain the proper degree of restriction. An inappropriately adjusted band leads to ineffective weight loss. As with the evolution of the technique of LAGB placement and the reduction in late complications, substantial changes in postoperative band management have contributed to improved weight loss.

Patients are discharged on a liquid diet for 2 weeks, which is transitioned to soft and pureed foods. Solid foods are prohibited to avoid emesis or feelings of undue fullness while the band settles into position and a pseudocapsule develops around the band [18]. Solid foods are initiated at 6 weeks. Feelings of satiety with small volumes of food are best achieved with solids. Softer foods and calorie-containing liquids are avoided. Patients are instructed to begin a graduated exercise program at discharge.

Initially, band adjustments were performed routinely with fluoroscopic guidance as needed based on weight loss, using the rate of contrast flow through the stoma as a guide for calibration. The frequency of adjustments was variable, often left to the patient's discretion. In the absence of established guidelines for band management, reported weight loss varied considerably among published series. A band adjusted too tightly leads to an aversion of solid foods, the ingestion of higher-calorie liquids and softer foods, and poor weight loss. Underappreciation of this observation often resulted in further tightening of the band. Poor weight loss, a high incidence of gastroesophageal reflux and esophageal dilation, pouch enlargement with obstruction, and frequent band extirpation were reported in several series [19,20].

Adjustments should be performed only after evaluating the patient's weight loss, eating habits, and symptoms. A rapid loss of satiety, increased meal volume, and increasing hunger between meals are indications for adding fluid. Vomiting, reflux, heartburn, and frequent consumption of softer foods suggest the band is too tight. Adjustments can be performed easily in the office without the need for radiographic evaluation [18]. Although relying on clinical symptoms, some authors find the additional information gained from a contrast study beneficial and continue to perform adjustments under fluoroscopic guidance [21]. Patients should be evaluated every 4 to 6 weeks during the first postoperative year. Gradual weight loss, 0.5 to 1 kg/wk, is the goal. Shen and colleagues [22] have demonstrated that, unlike gastric bypass, weight loss after LAGB is dependent upon frequent follow-up, at 1 year, patients who had returned for more than six visits had excess weight loss (EWL) of 50%, compared with only 42% EWL in patients who had six or fewer visits [22].

Results of laparoscopic adjustable gastric banding—perioperative complications

A major advantage of the LAGB is its safety. An evidence-based review by the Australian Safety and Efficacy Register of New Interventional Procedures-Surgical found that LAGB was associated with a median overall morbidity rate of 11.3% with a mean short-term mortality of 0.05%, compared with a 23.6% morbidity and 0.5% mortality for RYGB [10]. Major perioperative complications are infrequent with LAGB. O'Brien and colleagues [13], in a series of 1065 patients including their initial experience with perigastric placement and the later pars flaccida approach, reported a 1.5% incidence of perioperative complications delaying discharge or requiring readmission. Complications included port site infection in 0.9%, early obstruction in 0.38%, and symptomatic deep venous thrombosis in

0.09%. There were no perioperative deaths. Chevallier and colleagues [23], in 1000 LAGB placed by perigastric and pars flaccida techniques, reported four gastroesophageal perforations (0.4%) of which two were recognized intraoperatively, early prolapse in 0.3%, pulmonary embolism in 0.2%, and acute respiratory distress syndrome in 0.2%. There were 12 conversions to an open procedure (10 in the first 50 cases) and no mortalities [23]. Weiner and colleagues [24], in 984 LAGB reported one gastric perforation in a patient with prior hiatal surgery and one early prolapse. There were no mortalities or conversions to an open procedure. Fielding and colleagues [25], reporting 335 cases placed by the perigastric technique, reported two reoperations for improper band positioning, one subphrenic abscess, and four wound infections requiring antibiotic therapy, with no mortalities.

Similar results have been published in contemporary series in the United States using the pars flaccida technique. Spivak and colleagues [26], in 271 patients, reported a 1.8% incidence of acute obstruction, one pulmonary embolism, and one trocar-site hemorrhage. Open conversion was required in three patients (1.1%), one of which occurred during simultaneous laparoscopic cholecystectomy after successful band placement. There were no mortalities. Mean operative time was 42 minutes, and mean hospital stay was 1 day. Ren and colleagues [27], in a two-institution experience with 445 patients, reported a 2.7% incidence of early obstruction, conversion for bleeding requiring splenectomy in one patient (0.2%), and a single mortality. Post-mortem examination revealed no cause of death. Mean length of hospital stay was 1.1 days.

Acute obstruction caused by outlet stenosis may be seen after pars flaccida placement of the Lap-Band. Shen and Ren [28] reported that removal of large perigastric fat pads reduced the incidence of early stomal obstruction from 8% (11/143) to 0% in 124 patients. Five of 11 early obstructions were managed by laparoscopic revision. Alternatively, early obstruction, after excluding prolapse, may be managed conservatively. Eliminating oral intake while waiting for resolution of perioperative edema avoids the need for reoperation in the majority of patients.

Although life-threatening perioperative complications are less frequent after LAGB than after laparoscopic RYGB, LAGB placement does require advanced laparoscopic skills. Higher complication rates have been reported in smaller series. Although LAGB placement is technically simpler than laparoscopic RYGB, a learning curve does exist. Shapiro and colleagues, despite advanced laparoscopic experience, noted significant reductions in operative time (79 versus 59 minutes) and early and late complications (37% versus 7%) when comparing the first 30 patients with the second 30 patients [29].

Results of laparoscopic adjustable gastric banding—late complications

The evolution of the technique of LAGB placement from the perigastric to the pars flaccida technique has greatly reduced the incidence of gastric prolapse, pouch dilatation, and erosion. Weiner and colleagues [24] reported a prolapse rate of 5.3% with the perigastric technique (17% in the first 100 patients), which was reduced to 0.2% with the pars flaccida technique. The incidence of erosion was 0.3%. Minor port-related complications occurred in 2.5%. No band extirpations were required in the 407 bands placed using the pars flaccida technique. Chevalier and colleagues [23] noted a reduction in the incidence of prolapse from 24% with the perigastric approach (91/378) to 2% with pars flaccida placement (13/622). Band erosion was detected in 0.3%, and 5.7% required port revision. O'Brien and Dixon [13], in a series of 1150 LAGB, reported a 31% rate of prolapse in their first 400 patients, 12% in the second 400 patients, and 3% in the last 350 patients treated. The incidence of erosion was 3.2%, all occurring in the first 500 patients. Dargent [30] compared the rate of prolapse in 511 LAGB placed by the perigastric technique with 462 patients subsequently undergoing LAGB by the pars flaccida approach, noting a decrease from 6.2% to 0.6%.

The improved results with the pars flaccida technique may be confounded by surgeon experience and length of follow-up. The rate of reoperations increases with longer follow-up, and LAGB with the pars flaccida approach were performed later in the surgeons' experience. O'Brien and Dixon [31] therefore performed a randomized, controlled trial comparing the perigastric and pars flaccida techniques. The rate of prolapse was significantly reduced with the pars flaccida technique (3% versus 10%, $P < .04$).

Late complications are comparable in United States series using the pars flaccida technique. In 445 patients, Ren and colleagues reported a prolapse rate of 3.1%, erosion in 0.2%, and port-related complications in 3% [27]. Two bands were removed for intra-abdominal abscesses at 2 and 3 months postoperatively. No cases of esophageal dilatation were observed. The overall incidence of band removal was 0.9%. Spivak and colleagues [26] reported a 1.8% incidence of prolapse, and a 7.3% incidence of minor port related complications; 6.6% of patients had gastric pouch dilation or esophageal dilation, which resolved with band deflation. There were no erosions or band removals. In a cohort of 207 patients who had diabetes, hypertension, or both with at least 1-ear follow-up, Ponce and colleagues [32] reported a prolapse rate of 3%, port infections in 2.4% (compared with an overall rate of 0.97% in all patients who had 1-year follow-up), erosion in 0.5%, and band removal in 1%.

It is apparent that the technique of band placement must be considered when evaluating late complication rates in reports of LAGB. Studies using the perigastric technique are of historical interest only. Contemporary results with the pars flaccida technique yield prolapse rates lower than 5%, erosions in fewer than 1%, port-related complications in 2% to 6%, and band extirpations in less than 3% of patients undergoing LAGB. Esophageal dilatation occurs only with overtightening of the band in response to fluid removal or with prolapse and is reported infrequently.

Life-threatening late complications after LAGB are infrequent. Almost all may be managed laparoscopically or by a local outpatient procedure. Erosions usually present insidiously, with failure of weight loss or port-site infection. Laparoscopic removal is standard. Although not advocated by most authors, O'Brien and Dixon [13] have reported simultaneous replacement of the Lap-Band at the time of removal for erosion in 12 patients without complication. Prolapse, which presents with symptoms of progressive reflux, vomiting, and dysphagia not responding to band deflation, may be readily diagnosed by an upper-gastrointestinal series. Laparoscopic repositioning or replacement is successful in most cases. Port disconnection or leakage can be managed as a local outpatient procedure. Introduction of a redesigned port seems to have decreased the frequency of this complication. Port-site infections may be minimized by perioperative antibiotic administration [24] and by sing proper aseptic techniques during band adjustment. After excluding band erosion, port infections are managed by removal of the port, dropping the band tubing back into the peritoneal cavity. After resolution of the local infection and wound healing, the port is replaced at a remote site, laparoscopically retrieving the tubing.

Weight loss following laparoscopic adjustable gastric banding

Weight loss after LAGB clearly depends on proper band adjustments and a frequent adjustment schedule during the first 1 to 2 years postoperatively. The need for frequent adjustments results from the loss of perigastric fat within the band with weight loss, loosening the band and permitting increased intake. Weight loss after LAGB is significantly slower than after RYGB, so comparisons between the operations demonstrate superior weight loss with RYGB when only early results are reported. Potential benefits of the gradual weight loss observed with LAGB include a reduced incidence of nutritional deficiencies, hair loss, and cholelithiasis.

Vertruyen [33] reported 543 LAGB patients (mean preoperative BMI, 44) with 96% follow-up at a median of 36 months. Percent EWL was 38% at 12 months, 61% at 24 months, and 62% at 36 months. Weight loss was maintained at greater than 50% EWL for as long as 7 years. Bands were removed in 14 patients (2.6%), 6 of whom had maintained ideal body weight. Weiner and colleagues [24] reported an 8-year percent EWL of 59.3% in their first 100 LAGB patients who had perigastric placement (97% follow-up). If the five patients requiring band removal were included, percent EWL fell to 54%. Belachew and colleagues [34] reported 763 patients (mean preoperative BMI, 42) with a 90% follow-up at a minimum of 4 years. Percent EWL was 40% at 12 months, 50% at 24 months, and ranged between 50% and 60% at 48 months and beyond; 3.1% of patients required band removal. Angrisani and colleagues [35] from the Italian

Collaborative Study Group for Lap-Band System registry, reported a 54.8% EWL in 381 of 573 patients who had LAGB placed with 5-year follow-up. Twenty-seven percent were lost to follow-up, 5.7% underwent band removal, 1.9% were converted to other bariatric procedures, and 1.2% died of unrelated causes. Dargent [36], in 500 LAGB placed with greater than 99% follow-up, reported 56% EWL at 1 year, 65% at 2 years, and 64% at 3 years. Band removal was required in 1%. O'Brien and colleagues [37] also reported excellent long-term results in 709 patients who underwent LAGB. Mean BMI was 45. Follow-up was 98.6%. Percent EWL was 47% at 1 year (492 patients), 53% at 2 years (336 patients), 53% at 3 years (273 patients), 52% at 4 years (112 patients), 54% at 5 years (32 patients), and 57% at 6 years (10 patients). Fewer than 2% had bands removed. These studies demonstrate excellent long-term results with the Lap-Band, with a mean EWL greater than 50% at 5 years and beyond. This experience compares favorably with the long-term results after RYGB [38,39].

Because of high complication rates and poor weight loss in initial reports of LAGB in the United States [19,40], it has been suggested that cultural and dietary differences make LAGB less suitable in Americans than in international populations. Perigastric placement and inadequate adjustment protocols contributed to these disappointing early results; contemporary series from the United States demonstrate results comparable to those of foreign series. Fox and colleagues [41] reported 105 patients (mean BMI, 46.7) who had LAGB placed in Mexico but were followed in a Tacoma, Washington clinic. Percent EWL was 61.1% at 1 year (50 patients), 74.8% at 2 years (35 patients), and 72.4% at 3 years (23 patients). Rubenstein and colleagues [42] reported their experience with 63 patients in the FDA B trial. All bands were placed with the perigastric technique. Mean percent EWL was 38.3% at 1 year, 46.6% at 2 years, and 53.6% at 3 years. Spivak and colleagues [26], in a cohort of 271 patients (mean BMI, 45.3), reported EWL of 40% at 12 months and 43% at 24 months. Ren and colleagues [27], in a multi-institutional report of early results, documented a 44.3% EWL at 1 year in 99 patients (mean preoperative BMI, 52.7). Ponce and colleagues [32] reported results in 413 patients (mean BMI, 46.2) with at least 1 year follow-up, demonstrating 41.2% EWL at 1 year (402 patients, 97.3% follow-up) and 63.3% at 2 years (91 patients, 94.8% follow-up). Jan and colleagues [43] compared weight loss in 154 LAGB patients (mean BMI, 50.9; mean age, 46 years) with 219 patients undergoing laparoscopic RYGB (mean BMI, 49.5; mean age, 42 years) between October 2000 and November 2003. EWL for LAGB and RYGB, respectively, was 36% versus 64% at 1 year, 45% versus 70% at 2 years, and 60% versus 57% at 3 years. As expected, weight loss was more rapid after gastric bypass, but the difference diminished considerably by 3 years because LAGB patients continued to lose weight whereas RYGB patients often had weight regain. At the University of Texas Southwestern Medical Center at Dallas, we placed 327 Lap-Bands (mean preoperative BMI, 49.2) from November 2001 through August 2004, with excellent early weight loss through September 2004 of 44% at 1 year and 61% at 2 years. Bands have been removed in 2.7% of patients.

These results demonstrate that, with the pars flaccida technique and appropriate band adjustments, LAGB is effective in Americans. The belief that Americans are different when it comes to weight-loss surgery and the LAGB seems to be a fallacy.

Laparoscopic adjustable gastric banding in special populations

The massively obese

The ability to place a band laparoscopically in the massively superobese offers significant advantages in terms of perioperative morbidity and mortality compared with conventional open surgery. Although laparoscopic RYGB has been reported in the superobese, it is technically much more demanding. The increased risk of major perioperative complications with gastric bypass in patients in whom diagnostic imaging often is not possible complicates management. Although it has been suggested that LAGB is not as successful in the superobese, available data do not support this theory. Fielding [44] reported 76 patients who had a BMI of 60 or higher (median BMI, 69; range, 60–104) undergoing LAGB. There were no mortalities, and median hospital stay was 3 days. Six patients had prior VBG, five of whom subsequently required band removal for dysphagia. Fielding currently does not advocate LAGB as a revisional procedure for failed gastroplasties. Of the remaining 70 patients, 69 bands remain in place. EWL was 46.7% at 1 year, 56.6% at 2 years, 59.1% at 3 years, 60.4% at 4 years, and 61.4% at 5 years. More than 80% of patients maintained more than 50% EWL at all time points 2 years and beyond. In the series by Fox and colleagues [41] of Americans having LAGB in Mexico, 35 of the 100 patients were superobese (BMI ≥50). Percent EWL was 52.8% at 1 year, 67.5% at 2 years, and 65.8% at 3 years. These results compare favorably with the weight loss observed with RYGB [38] and long-limb RYGB [45].

Extremes of age

With the aging of the population, the number of older patients seeking weight-loss surgery is increasing. Although there are clear benefits in quality of life and improvement in comorbid illness, improvements in longevity are less than in the younger population. Because increasing age has been demonstrated to be a major risk factor for mortality after gastric bypass [46], the reduced perioperative risk associated with LAGB makes it an attractive option in the older morbidly obese patient. Nehoda and colleagues [47] reported 68 patients age 50 years or older undergoing LAGB, with results and complications comparable with those in the younger cohort. One erosion in the older group required endoscopic removal, and one band was replaced for leakage (Swedish Adjustable Gastric Band, Ethicon Endosurgery,

Cincinnati, Ohio). EWL was 68% at 12 months and 71% at 24 months. We have placed 60 LAGB in patients aged 60 years and older (mean age, 65 years; range, 60–76 years) without mortality. Although the incidence of prolapse and band extirpation has been higher than in the younger cohort, weight loss and reduction of comorbidities have been excellent.

Adolescents

The prevalence of overweight in the pediatric population in the United States has tripled during the last 30 years, and obesity-related conditions previously associated with adults such as hypertension, dyslipidemia, type 2 diabetes, and obstructive sleep apnea are becoming increasingly more prevalent in the pediatric age group. A recent consensus statement has established guidelines for bariatric surgery in adolescents [48]. Criteria include

Attainment of physiologic maturity
A BMI of 40 or higher with serious obesity-related comorbidities or a
    BMI of 50 or higher with less severe comorbidities
Demonstrated decisional capacity
A supportive family environment

Lower perioperative morbidity and mortality, gradual weight loss with few nutritional complications, and reversibility make LAGB an appealing bariatric procedure in the overweight adolescent. Widhalm and colleagues [49] reported results of LAGB in eight adolescents (mean BMI, 49.1). There were no perioperative or late complications with short-term follow-up. At a mean follow-up of only 10 months, mean weight loss was 25 kg, or approximately 32.3% excess BMI lost. Dolan and Fielding [50] reported 17 adolescents (mean BMI, 42.2), aged 12 to 19 years, with a median follow-up of 25 months. There were no major perioperative complications. Late reoperations were required in two patients. One required laparoscopic repositioning of a prolapsed band; the second required replacement of a leaking port. EWL was 49.2% at 1 year and 69.3% at 2 years. More than 80% of adolescents had EWL of 50% or more by 24 months after surgery. Although experience is limited, as is experience with all bariatric surgical procedures in this age group, LAGB seems to be a safe and effective method for weight loss for obese adolescents. LAGB in adolescents should be performed only in a multidisciplinary weight-loss management program with providers experienced in meeting the unique physical and psychologic needs of the adolescent.

**Laparoscopic adjustable gastric banding in the obese
(body mass index 30–35)**

The current guidelines for weight loss surgery (BMI ≥ 40 or ≥ 35 with comorbidities) were established by the National Institutes of Health consensus panel based on available evidence regarding the risks and benefits of surgery for obesity weighed against the risks of morbid obesity [16]. Since 1991, substantial knowledge has been gained regarding the health risks of morbid obesity. In addition, improvements in the safety and efficacy of bariatric surgery have been demonstrated. As a result, it has been suggested that the minimum weight requirements for obesity surgery be lowered. Angrisani and colleagues [51], for the Italian Collaborative Study Group for Lap-Band System, reported 210 patients who had a BMI of 35 or lower undergoing LAGB as a primary weight loss procedure. There were no perioperative complications. Late complications included six pouch dilations or prolapse requiring reoperation, two erosions, and four port complications. Eight bands were removed for complications (0.3%), including one removed for psychologic intolerance. EWL was 52.5% at 1 year, 61.3% at 2 years, 64.7% at 3 years, 68.8% at 4 years, and 71.9% at 5 years. Major comorbidities were present in only a few of the patients, with diabetes resolving in four of four patients and hypertension resolving in eight of nine patients. O'Brien and colleagues [52] reported a randomized, controlled trial of optimal medical therapy versus LAGB in 79 patients who had a BMI between 30 and 35. There were no perioperative complications in the 39 patients randomly assigned to surgical therapy. Reoperation was required for prolapse in two patients. Weight loss at 2 years was 71.5% EWL in the surgical group compared with 21.4% EWL in the controls ($P < .001$). LAGB resulted in significantly greater improvement in quality of life and all measures of the metabolic syndrome. Although primary bariatric procedures cannot currently be recommended for patients who have a BMI lower than 35 outside of institutional review board–approved protocols, the safety and controlled weight loss of the LAGB make it an ideal procedure for this population.

Resolution of comorbidities with laparoscopic adjustable gastric banding

Weight loss is a benefit of bariatric surgery, but improvements in comorbid illness and quality of life are the primary goals. Type 2 diabetes mellitus is a major contributor to the long-term morbidity associated with morbid obesity. Dolan and colleagues [53] reported that 65% of 49 diabetics with at least 6 months follow-up no longer required any diabetes medications after LAGB. Dixon and O'Brien [54] demonstrated normalization of glucose, hemoglobin A_{1c}, and insulin resistance in 64% of type 2 diabetics and improvement in an additional 26% after LAGB. Ponce and colleagues [32], in a North American population undergoing LAGB, reported resolution of diabetes in 66% of diabetics at 1 year, increasing to 80% at 2 years as EWL increased from 39.2% to 52.6%. Hypertension resolved in 74% of patients at 2 years. O'Brien and Dixon [13] noted resolution or improvement on hypertension in 92% of patients undergoing LAGB. LAGB has also been demonstrated to improve lipid profiles, asthma, sleep apnea, menstrual irregularities and infertility, depression, joint and back pain, stress incontinence, self-esteem, and overall quality of life [13,37,55].

Early reports of an increased rate of gastroesophageal reflux (GERD) after LAGB [19] and an increased incidence of prolapse in patients who have hiatal hernia [56] has led some to question LAGB placement in the presence of a hiatal hernia. Reflux after LAGB is usually an indication of an overly tightened band or a sign of prolapse or pouch dilatation, a complication greatly reduced by the adoption of the pars flaccida approach. O'Brien reported total resolution of GERD in 89% of LAGB patients, improvement in 5%, no change in 2.5%, and aggravation of symptoms in 2.5% [13]. Dolan and colleagues [57] reported 62 patients undergoing crural repair of hiatal hernia at the time of LAGB placement. With a median follow-up of 14 months, there was one prolapse requiring laparoscopic repositioning. Only six patients required antireflux medications postoperatively. LAGB is an effective therapy for the management of GERD.

Summary

More than 8 million persons in the United States have a BMI of 40 or higher, and an additional 23 million persons have a BMI between 35 and 40. Many of these persons have significant obesity-related comorbidities. Bariatric surgery remains the only effective treatment for morbid obesity. Despite the exponential increase in the number of weight-loss operations being performed, it is evident that, with 100,000 to 200,000 procedures performed annually, most patients suffering the complications of morbid obesity are not receiving the best available therapy. Although cost or lack of insurance coverage is a deterrent to many, many patients fail to seek surgical options because of fear of operative complications or death. LAGB provides a safer alternative, with an incidence of complications one half that after gastric bypass and one tenth the mortality [10]. Complications, unlike anastomotic leaks or intestinal obstruction, rarely are life threatening. Most are managed laparoscopically or by minor, outpatient procedures. Most importantly, weight loss has proven durable. Although long-term follow-up has yet to reach the 10-year mark, the number of published series and patients who have 5 years or more follow-up exceeds that of gastric bypass. Weight loss is comparable, at 50% to 60% EWL. Resolution of obesity-related comorbidities parallels the weight loss after LAGB. Despite initial reports, with refinements in surgical and band management techniques, results from centers in the United States are comparable with those of the best international series. LAGB is a safe and effective option for the morbidly obese patient seeking weight-loss surgery.

References

[1] Hedley AA, Ogden CL, Johnson CL, et al. Prevalence of overweight and obesity among US children, adolescents, and adults, 1999–2002. JAMA 2004;291(23):2847–50.

[2] Calle EE, Thun MJ, Petrelli JM, et al. Body-mass index and mortality in a prospective cohort of US adults. N Engl J Med 1999;341:1097–105.

[3] Buchwald H, Avidor Y, Braunwald E, et al. Bariatric surgery: a systematic review and meta-analysis. JAMA 2004;292:1724–37.

[4] Christou NV, Sampalis JS, Liberman M. Surgery decreases long-term mortality, morbidity, and health care use in morbidly obese patients. Ann Surg 2004;240:416–24.

[5] Flum DR, Dellinger EP. Impact of gastric bypass operation on survival: a population-based analysis. J Am Coll Surg 2004;199:543–51.

[6] Mason EE. Vertical banded gastroplasty for obesity. Arch Surg 1982;117(5):701–6.

[7] Szinicz G, Schnapka G. A new method in the surgical treatment of disease. Acta Chir Aust 1982;14:Suppl 43.

[8] Kuzmak LI, Yap IS, Mcguire L, et al. Surgery for morbid obesity using an inflatable gastric band. AORN J 1990;51(5):1307–24.

[9] Belachew M, Legrand M, Defechereux T, et al. Laparoscopic adjustable silicon banding in the treatment of morbid obesity: a preliminary report. Surg Endosc 1994;8:1354–6.

[10] Chapman AE, Kiroff G, Game P, et al. Laparoscopic adjustable gastric banding in the treatment of obesity: a systematic literature review. Surgery 2004;135(3):326–51.

[11] Belachew M, Legrand M, Vincent V, et al. Laparoscopic placement of adjustable silicone gastric band in the treatment of morbid obesity: how to do it. Obes Surg 1995;5(1):66–70.

[12] Favretti F, Cardiere GB, Segato G, et al. Laparoscopic adjustable silicone gastric banding: technique and results. Obes Surg 1995;5(4):364–71.

[13] O'Brien PE, Dixon JB. Laparoscopic adjustable gastric banding in the treatment of morbid obesity. Arch Surg 2003;138(4):376–82.

[14] DeMaria EJ, Sugerman HJ. A critical look at laparoscopic adjustable silicone gastric banding for the treatment of morbid obesity: does it measure up? Surg Endosc 2000;14:697–9.

[15] Belachew M, Zimmermann J-M. Evolution of a paradigm for laparoscopic adjustable gastric banding. Am J Surg 2002;184:21S–5S.

[16] Consensus Development Conference Panel. Gastrointestinal surgery for severe obesity. Ann Intern Med 1991;115(12):956–61.

[17] Ren CJ, Fielding GA. Laparoscopic adjustable gastric banding: surgical technique. J Laparoenosc Adv Surg Tech A 2003;13(4):257–63.

[18] Favretti F, O'Brien PE, Dixon JB. Patient management after Lap-Band placement. Am J Surg 2002;184:38S–41S.

[19] DeMaria EJ, Sugerman HJ, Meador JG, et al. High failure rate after laparoscopic adjustable silicone gastric banding for treatment of morbid obesity. Ann Surg 2001;233(6):809–18.

[20] Niville E, Dams A. Late pouch dilation after laparoscopic adjustable gastric banding: incidence, treatment, and outcome. Obes Surg 1999;9:381–4.

[21] Cadiere GB, Himpens J, Vertuyen M, et al. Laparoscopic gastroplasty (adjustable silicone gastric banding). Semin Laparosc Surg 2000;7:55–65.

[22] Shen R, Dugay G, Rajaram K, et al. Impact of patient follow-up on weight loss after bariatric surgery. Obes Surg 2004;14:514–9.

[23] Chevallier J-M, Zinzindohoue F, Douard R, et al. Complications after laparoscopic adjustable gastric banding for morbid obesity: experience with 1,000 patients over 7 years. Obes Surg 2004;14:407–14.

[24] Weiner R, Blanco-Engert R, Weiner S, et al. Outcome after laparoscopic adjustable gastric banding—8 years experience. Obes Surg 2003;13:427–34.

[25] Fielding GA, Rhodes M, Nathanson LK. Laparoscopic gastric banding for morbid obesity: surgical outcome in 335 cases. Surg Endosc 1999;13(6):550–4.

[26] Spivak H, Anwar F, Burton S, et al. The Lap-Band system in the United States: one surgeon's experience with 271 patients. Surg Endosc 2004;18:198–202.

[27] Ren CJ, Weiner M, Allen JW. Favorable early results of gastric banding for morbid obesity: the American experience. Surg Endosc 2004;18:543–6.

[28] Shen R, Ren CJ. Removal of peri-gastric fat prevents acute obstruction after Lap-Band surgery. Obes Surg 2004;14:224–9.

[29] Shapiro K, Patel S, Abdo Z, et al. Laparoscopic adjustable gastric banding: is there a learning curve? Surg Endosc 2004;18:48–50.

[30] Dargent J. Pouch dilatation and slippage after adjustable gastric banding: is it still an issue? Obes Surg 2003;13:111–5.

[31] O'Brien P, Dixon J. Pars flaccida versus perigastric pathways for the placement of the Lap-Band system [abstract 40]. Presented at the 20th Annual Meeting of the American Society for Bariatric Surgery. Boston, MA: 2003. Obes Surg 2003;13:211.

[32] Ponce J, Haynes B, Paynter S, et al. Effect of Lap-Band induced weight loss on type 2 diabetes mellitus and hypertension. Obes Surg 2004;14:1335–42.

[33] Vertruyen M. Experience with the Lap-Band system up to 7 years. Obes Surg 2002;12: 569–72.

[34] Belachew M, Belva PH, Desaive C. Long-term results of laparoscopic adjustable gastric banding for the treatment of morbid obesity. Obes Surg 2002;12(4):564–8.

[35] Angrisani L, DiLorenzo N, Favretti F, et al. The Italian group for Lap-Band: Predictive value of initial body mass index for weight loss after 5 years of follow-up. Surg Endosc 2004; 18:1524–7.

[36] Dargent J. Laparoscopic adjustable gastric banding: lessons from the first 500 patients in a single institution. Obes Surg 1999;9:446–52.

[37] O'Brien PE, Dixon JB, Brown W, et al. The laparoscopic adjustable gastric band (Lap-Band): a prospective study of medium-term effects on weight, health and quality of life. Obes Surg 2002;12:652–60.

[38] MacLean LD, Rhode BM, Nohr CW. Late outcome of isolated gastric bypass. Ann Surg 2000;231(4):524–8.

[39] Pories WJ, Swanson MS, MacDonald KG, et al. Who would have thought it? An operation proves to be the most effective therapy for adult-onset diabetes mellitus. Ann Surg 1995; 222(3):339–50.

[40] Doherty C, Maher JW, Heitshusen DS. Long-term data indicate a progressive loss in efficacy of adjustable silicone gastric banding for the surgical treatment of morbid obesity. Surgery 2002;132(4):724–8.

[41] Fox SR, Fox KM, Srikanth MS, et al. The Lap-Band system in a North American population. Obes Surg 2003;13:275–80.

[42] Rubenstein RB, Ferraro DR, Raffel J. Laparoscopic adjustable gastric banding at a US center with up to 3-year follow-up. Obes Surg 2002;12:380–4.

[43] Jan JC, Hong D, Pereira N, et al. Laparoscopic adjustable gastric banding versus laparoscopic gastric bypass for morbid obesity: a single-institution comparison study of early results. J Gastrointest Surg 2005;9(1):30–41.

[44] Fielding GA. Laparoscopic adjustable gastric banding for massive superobesity (> 60 body mass index kg/m^2). Surg Endosc 2003;17:1541–5.

[45] Brolin RE, Kenler HA, German JH, et al. Long-limb gastric bypass in the superobese: a prospective randomized study. Ann Surg 1992;215:387–95.

[46] Livingston EH, Huerta S, Arthur D, et al. Male gender is a predictor of morbidity and age is a predictor of mortality for patients undergoing gastric bypass surgery. Ann Surg 2002; 236(6):576–82.

[47] Nehoda H, Hourmont K, Sauper T, et al. Laparoscopic gastric banding in older patients. Arch Surg 2001;136:1171–6.

[48] Inge TH, Krebs NF, Garcia VF, et al. Bariatric surgery for severely overweight adolescents: concerns and recommendations. Pediatrics 2004;114(1):217–23.

[49] Widhalm K, Dietrich S, Prager G. Adjustable gastric banding surgery in morbidly obese adolescents: experiences with eight patients. Int J Obes 2004;28:S42–5.

[50] Dolan K, Fielding G. A comparison of laparoscopic adjustable gastric banding in adolescents and adults. Surg Endosc 2004;18:45–7.

[51] Angrisani L, Favretti F, Furbetta F, et al. Italian Group for Lap-Band System: results of multicenter study on patients with BMI $\leq$ 35 kg/m^2. Obes Surg 2004;14:415–8.

[52] O'Brien P, Dixon J, Laurie C. The management of obesity: a prospective randomized controlled trial (RCT) of medical versus surgical therapy [abstract 3]. Presented at the 21st Annual Meeting of the American Society for Bariatric Surgery. San Diego, California. June 12–18, 2004.

[53] Dolan K, Bryant R, Fielding G. Treating diabetes in the morbidly obese by laparoscopic gastric banding. Obes Surg 2003;13:439–43.

[54] Dixon JB, O'Brien PE. Health outcomes of severely obese type 2 diabetic subjects 1 year after laparoscopic adjustable gastric banding. Diabetes Care 2002;25(2):358–63.

[55] Frigg A, Peterli R, Peters T. Reduction in co-morbidities 4 years after laparoscopic adjustable gastric banding. Obes Surg 2004;14:216–23.

[56] Greenstein RJ, Nissan A, Jaffin B. Esophageal anatomy and function in laparoscopic gastric restrictive bariatric surgery: implications for patient selection. Obes Surg 1998;8:199–206.

[57] Dolan K, Finch R, Fielding G. Laparoscopic gastric banding and crural repair in the obese patient with a hiatal hernia. Obes Surg 2003;13:772–5.

ELSEVIER
SAUNDERS

SURGICAL
CLINICS OF
NORTH AMERICA

Surg Clin N Am 85 (2005) 807–817

Long Limb Roux en Y Gastric Bypass Revisited

Robert E. Brolin, MD[a,b,*]

[a]*University of Pittsburgh Medical Center, 200 Lothrop Street, Pittsburgh,*
PA 15213-2582, USA
[b]*University Medical Center at Princeton, 253 Witherspoon Street, Princeton, NJ 08540, USA*

In the early era of Roux en Y gastric bypass (RYGB), Roux limb length typically was in the range of 50 cm to 75 cm and rarely exceeded 100 cm [1–3]. In that era, Roux limb length was focused on elimination of bile reflux. In our early experience with RYGB, when using a 50-cm to 75-cm Roux limb, many of the heaviest patients failed to achieve satisfactory weight loss postoperatively. This observation led us to design a prospective randomized clinical study to learn whether a modest increase in Roux limb length would improve weight loss results without producing a higher incidence of metabolic and other complications. In our prospective randomized study, a 150-cm Roux limb was compared with a conventional 75-cm Roux limb in 45 patients. The 150-cm measurement was chosen arbitrarily and dubbed "long limb." This modification is illustrated in Fig. 1. Gastric pouch volume was the same in both groups. Because weight loss results generally were satisfactory in less obese patients when using a 50- to 75-cm limb RYGB, we restricted our protocol to super obese patients who weighed at least 200 pounds more than their ideal body weight according to standard life insurance tables [4]. We used the number of pounds overweight in our selection of patients because body mass index (BMI) was not a commonly used weight measurement in 1984 when the first patient was entered into our prospective study. Extending Roux limb length beyond 100 cm was not evaluated carefully before the publication of the results of our prospective study in 1992 [5].

* NJBariatrics, 4250 U.S. Route 1 North, Suite 1, Monmouth Junction, NJ 08852.
E-mail address: rbrolin@njbariatricspc.com

0039-6109/05/$ - see front matter © 2005 Elsevier Inc. All rights reserved.
doi:10.1016/j.suc.2005.03.003 *surgical.theclinics.com*

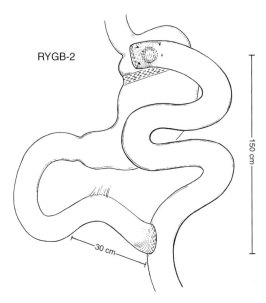

Fig. 1. Roux-en-Y gastric bypass in which the TA 90-B stapler (U.S. Surgical Corp., Norwalk, Connecticut) is fired across the cardia of the stomach to create a 20 ± 5 cm³ upper pouch. The jejunum is divided approximately 30 cm distal to the ligament of Treitz with the distal end anastomosed to the upper stomach using a circular stapler to create a 1.1-cm diameter anastomosis. The proximal end of the jejunum is anastomosed 150 cm below the gastro-jejunostomy. (*From* Brolin RE, Kenler HA, Gorman JG, et al. Long-limb gastric bypass in the super-obese: A prospective randomized study. Ann Surg 1992;215:388; with permission.)

What is long limb gastric bypass?

The patients who had a 150-cm Roux limb achieved significantly greater weight loss at 2 and 3 years postoperatively versus the group that had a 75-cm Roux limb (Fig. 2). Moreover, there was no difference in the incidence of metabolic or other complications between the two groups. These results prompted many bariatric surgeons to extend the length of the Roux limb in their patients; however, many surgeons did not follow our technique "to the letter" but rather used other measurements for the Roux and biliopancreatic limb.

Only a few surgeons have reported their results with longer Roux limbs. In 1991, Bruder et al [6] reported a series of 55 patients who had RYGB performed with a 45-cm or 90-cm Roux limb. The patients were matched by age and gender, but the comparison of limb lengths was not randomized. Although limb length in the longer limb group was double that of the patients who had short limbs, 90 cm is "short" by current standards. These investigators reported that mean excess weight loss was 6% greater in the longer Roux limb group after 6 months with no difference in diarrhea or nutritional complications between the two groups. A follow-up study was published by Freeman et al [7] in 1997. Roux limb length was extended to

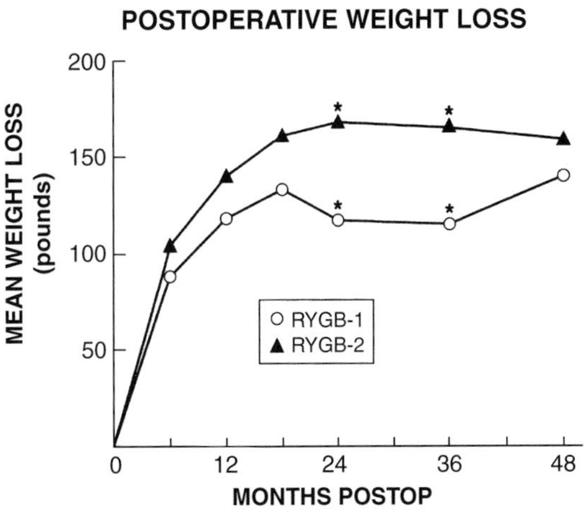

POSTOPERATIVE WEIGHT LOSS

Fig. 2. Weight loss in pounds through 4 years postoperatively. *Significant difference between the two groups ($P < 0.02$ by unpaired Student t test). (*From* Brolin RE, Kenler HA, Gorman JG, et al. Long-limb gastric bypass in the super-obese: A prospective randomized study. Ann Surg 1992;215:389; with permission.)

225 cm in a few patients, although the numbers of patients who had limb measurements at 225 cm or any other specific length was not stated in that report. Weight loss at 2 years postoperatively was substantially greater in the patients who had longer Roux limbs. There was no difference in metabolic sequelae between patients who had short and long limbs; however, several patients who had long limbs had "troublesome" diarrhea.

In 1997, Sugerman et al [8] reported a series of 22 superobese patients who failed to lose weight following conventional RYGB. They had revisional operations that incorporated a 140-cm Roux limb, a long unmeasured biliopancreatic limb, and a 150-cm common channel. This series followed a group of 5 patients who underwent RYGB with unsatisfactory weight loss who underwent a revisional RYGB that incorporated the same Roux limb measurement and a 50-cm common channel. All 5 patients developed severe protein calorie malnutrition with two late deaths secondary to hepatic failure. Sugerman's group concluded that biliopancreatic diversion that incorporated a small upper gastric pouch and a 50-cm common channel was unduly severe and could not be recommended. Conversely, the same procedure with a 150-cm common channel resulted in a mean loss of excess weight of 69% at 5 years postoperatively and manageable nutritional sequelae.

In 2000, MacLean et al [9] reported a significant difference in successful weight loss outcome following isolated RYGB between 96 superobese patients and 178 patients with a BMI of less than 50 kg/m^2. Although the superobese patients lost more weight than their less obese counterparts, their final mean BMI was 35 $\pm$ 7 kg/m^2. Moreover, 41 of the 96 superobese patients (43%) failed to lose 50% of their excess weight. All

274 patients were randomized in a short (40 cm) versus long (100 cm) Roux limb comparison [10]. MacLean et al also varied the length of the biliopancreatic limb (10 cm in the short limb group versus 100 cm in the long limb group). The superobese patients who had longer Roux and biliopancreatic limbs had significantly greater weight loss. Conversely, in the less obese patients (BMI < 50 kg/m^2) there was no difference in weight loss between the two groups. There also was no difference in the incidence of metabolic sequelae.

In 2001, Choban and Flancbaum [11] reported the results of a prospective, randomized comparison of three Roux limb lengths in 133 patients, including a 75-cm versus 150-cm limb length in 69 patients with a BMI of up to 50 kg/m^2. Sixty-four superobese patients were randomized to receive Roux limbs of 150 cm or 250 cm. Gastric pouch volume and length of the biliopancreatic limb were the same in all patients. In the less obese patients, the difference in limb length had no impact on postoperative weight loss. Conversely, the superobese patients who had 250-cm Roux limbs had significantly greater weight loss compared with the patients who had 150-cm limbs at 18 months postoperatively. This difference seemed to persist beyond 18 months but lost statistical significance as the number of patients that was available for follow-up decreased over time. The relative incidence of nutritional deficiencies was not addressed in this study.

In 2003, Feng et al [12] compared Roux limb lengths in 58 patients who underwent laparoscopic RYGB. The short Roux limb group included 45 patients who had lengths that ranged from 45 cm to 100 cm, whereas the limbs were 150 cm in remaining 13 patients. In this study, the difference in weight loss between the short and long limb groups was not significant; however, the number of patients that had long limbs was small and the mean BMI for the entire series was 44 kg/m^2. Nonetheless, a "trend toward an increased portion of patients with >50% excess weight loss ($P = 0.07$) was observed in the extended Roux limb group." This trend might have achieved statistical significance if more patients who had long limbs were included in this study.

In 2002, we reported the results of a 10-year evaluation of a "distal" RYGB in which the Roux enteroenterostomy was performed at 75 cm above the ileocecal junction [13]. This distal RYGB incorporated a 15-cm to 25-cm biliopancreatic limb and an upper gastric pouch with a capacity of up to 30 cm^3. Forty-eight superobese patients with a mean BMI of 68 kg/m^2, who had the distal RYGB were compared retrospectively with superobese patients who had "short" (50–75 cm) and "long" (150 cm) Roux limbs. Figs. 3 and 4 show weight loss expressed in pounds and BMI units through 5 years postoperatively. There were significant differences in weight loss among the three groups that began at 6 months postoperatively and persisted throughout the study. Greater weight loss was associated consistently with progressively longer Roux limb lengths. The duration of weight loss before stabilization also correlated with limb length. The short

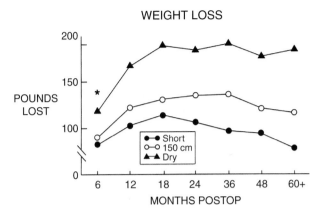

Fig. 3. Weight loss in pounds through 5 years postoperatively. There were significant differences between each of the three groups at at least 1 year postoperatively. *Significant difference between the short limb group and distal RY gastric bypass (D-RY) and 150-cm patients at 6 months postoperatievly (*P* < 0.05 by ANOVA with Student-Newman-Keuls test). (*From* Brolin RE, Lamarca LB, Kenler HA, et al. Malabsorptive gastric bypass in patients with super obesity. J Gastrointest Surg 2002;6:198; with permission.)

limb group stabilized between 12 and 18 months, whereas the patients who had 150-cm limbs or distal RYGB stabilized at 24 and 36 months, respectively. The percentage of weight that was regained from the mean time of stabilization was the same in patients who had short limbs and 150-cm limbs. Less weight was regained following distal malabsorptive RYGB; this

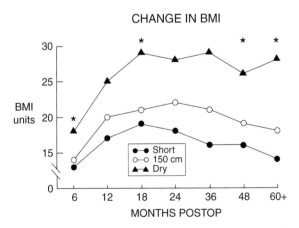

Fig. 4. Change in BMI through 5 years postoperatively. There were significant differences between each of the groups at 12, 24, and 36 months postoperatively. *Significant difference between the Dry patients and the shorter limb groups noted at 6, 18, 48, and 60 months (*P* < 0.05; by ANOVA with Student-Newman-Keuls test). (*From* Brolin RE, Lamarca LB, Kenler HA, et al. Malabsorptive gastric bypass in patients with super obesity. J Gastrointest Surg 2002;6:199; with permission.)

suggests that the malabsorptive component may contribute to long-term weight maintenance. Variability in eating behavior among individual patients is likely the most important factor in weight loss maintenance following bariatric operations. The incidence of metabolic problems was significantly greater following distal RYGB (Table 1).

In 1998, the Mayo Clinic group reported their experience with a very very long Roux limb in 26 superobese patients; the mean BMI was 67 ± 3 kg/m^2 [14]. Roux limb length was unmeasured; however, the common channel between the enteroenterostomy and the ileocecal junction was constant at 100 cm. At 2 years, the mean percentage of excess weight loss was 57%, which was less than the 64% mean excess weight loss that was observed in our patients who underwent a distal RYGB. The incidence of postoperative nutritional problems was not mentioned in the Mayo report.

In the early era of bariatric surgery there was only one current procedural terminology (CPT) code for RYGB. In 1994, a second CPT code for RYGB, #43847, was approved. This coding change distinguished short- and long-limb RYGB. CPT #43846 is described as "gastric restrictive procedure, with gastric bypass for morbid obesity; with short limb (less than 100 cm) Roux-en-Y gastroenterostomy." CPT #43847 is described as "gastric restrictive procedure, with gastric bypass for morbid obesity with small intestine reconstruction to limit absorption" [15]. Although a limb measurement is not listed for #43847, it is de facto that any limb measurement that exceeds 100 cm must be assigned this code because there are only two codes listed for RYGB!

Determination of experimental and investigative procedures

Several major insurance carriers deny coverage for any RYGB that is coded under #43847 on the basis that all procedures that are submitted under this code are "experimental or investigative." One major carrier's definition of "experimental/investigative" is an "intervention" that is "not proven to be as safe or effective in achieving an outcome equal to or

Table 1
Postoperative metabolic deficiencies

Operation	Iron	B-12	Anemia	Vit A	Vit D	Calcium	Albumin
Short (N = 80)	42 (52%)	30 (37%)	33 (41%)	_[a]	_[a]	_[a]	_[a]
150 cm (N = 102)	46 (45%)	34 (33%)	36 (35%)	_[a]	_[a]	_[a]	_[a]
D-RY (N = 39)	19 (49%)	3 (8%)[b]	36 (74%)[b]	4 (10%)	20 (51%)	4 (10%)	5 (13%)

[a] Not measured.

[b] Significant difference between D-RY patients and the other two groups. (Less than 0.003 by chi square test).

From Brolin RE, Lamarca LB, Kenler HA, et al. Malabsorptive gastric bypass in patients with super obesity. J Gastrointest Surg 2002;6:201; with permission.

exceeding the outcome of alternative therapies," or "does not improve health outcomes," or "does not permit conclusions concerning the effect of the interventions on health outcomes," or "is not proven to be applicable outside the research setting." The author recently submitted a request for approval of RYGB, CPT #43847 to be performed in a middle-aged woman (BMI = 63 kg/m^2) who had refractory hypertension, type II diabetes, sleep apnea, and degenerative arthritis. The carrier's denial included their criteria for "experimental/investigative" procedures as detailed above. The author appealed the denial and cited our 1992 prospective randomized study and MacLean et al's [10] 2001 report as evidence to refute the criteria in their denial letter. Not surprisingly, a second denial was received based upon their previously cited criteria without comment on the data in our 1992 paper or MacLean et al's report. A subsequent conversation with one of the carrier's medical directors was nonproductive. The medical director cited a recent "in-house" review of available bariatric surgical procedures that totally ignored our 1992 study and our more recent publication with longer follow-up [13]. Rather than continue with an apparently losing battle, this patient consented to have a less than 100-cm Roux limb gastric bypass which proceeded uneventfully.

It seems likely that the deepest root of the authorization problem for long-limb RYGB is the current descriptions of the two existing CPT codes. CPT #43846 and #43847 were approved for use more than 10 years ago. All of the prospective studies that confirmed the safety and efficacy of the long-limb RYGB that was described in our 1992 report were published during the past 5 years [10–12]. Unfortunately, CPT #43847 has lumped the 150-cm RYGB with the very very long limb/distal RYGB, which were introduced as malabsorptive procedures. All of the available data on the 150-cm RYGB show it to be as safe as an up to 100-cm RYGB in terms of complications, and more effective in producing weight loss. Conversely, the distal RYGB with a very (very) long Roux limb and an up to 150-cm common channel seems to produce better weight loss than the 150-cm RYGB, but at a defined metabolic price in terms of a greater variety and increased incidence of nutritional sequelae [8,13]. Although some degree of biliopancreatic diversion is inherent in RYGB, the degree of diversion that is likely to result in fat soluble vitamin deficiency and steatorrhea remains undetermined. There are sufficient data to justify the position that RYGB with a 150-cm Roux limb does not result in more metabolic sequelae than conventional short-limb RYGB [10,13].

Another factor that must be considered in the authorization process for bariatric operations is the motivation of individual insurance carriers. Fischer [16] recently recounted his experience as a member of the medical advisory panel (MAP) for the Technology Evaluation Center (TEC) which represents a "joint effort between the Kaiser Permanente Foundation and the Blue Cross and Blue Shield Association." Fischer commented that the TEC panel had difficulty believing that bariatric surgery improved "net health outcome." Moreover, he recounted that patients "often" regain their weight "sometimes needing a second procedure if they are not followed rigorously in a program with long term nutritional counseling." He later commented that no American study showed that gastric bypass resulted in improvement in "net health outcome." This conclusion flies in the face of hundreds of papers that showed dramatic improvement in all of the comorbidities that are associated with severe obesity following successful weight loss surgery. Fischer did not define "net health outcome" in his report. An important note in Fischer's commentary was that "the staff" of the insurance carriers collected all of the papers for review by the MAP and already had "whittled down" the collection to "prospective studies" by the time of presentation to the MAP. Our 1992 prospective randomized study apparently was not reviewed by the MAP. As a cynic regarding the motivations of health insurance carriers, the author seriously questions how or why the staff could not find at least one American study that showed improvement in "net health outcome" following bariatric surgery.

The TEC report prompted Horizon Blue Cross Blue Shield of New Jersey to deny CPT code #43847, after covering this code since its inception. In their justification for denial, long-limb gastric bypass is described as a "malabsorptive" procedure which has "the potential complications similar to those of the biliopancreatic bypass." Coding problems notwithstanding, it seems that denial is the primary agenda here.

In 2005 several new CPT codes for bariatric operations were approved for general use including separate codes for laparoscopic and open procedures. Among the new codes is a change in the descriptor for CPT #43846 to acknowledge an up to 150-cm Roux limb as "short." Justification for this change is the absence of data which show that a 150-cm limb produces more malabsorptive manifestations than shorter Roux limb measurements.

Very (very) long Roux limbs and biliopancreatic diversion

Cynicism aside, none of the malabsorptive modifications of RYGB have been subjected to a randomized, prospective comparison with conventional short-limb RYGB, CPT #43846; however, the outcome of such a study seems predictable based upon the available data. Weight loss likely would be significantly greater with the more malabsorptive modifications of RYGB. There also is likely to be a significantly greater incidence of several metabolic deficiencies with more malabsorption (see Table 1). Improvements in obesity-related comorbidities would likely be greater with more weight loss, although short-term differences in comorbidity improvement between the two procedures may not be dramatic. Long-term weight maintenance might be better with more malabsorption, which could result in more sustained improvement of comorbidities. A comparison of revision rates also would be relevant because a substantial number of superobese patients that have conventional RYGB require revision for inadequate weight loss. Conversely, ongoing nutritional problems might be the leading cause for revision after malabsorptive RYGB. Only 1.6% of the author's more than 200 patients who underwent a distal RYGB have required revision for refractory nutritional deficiencies, although 3.8% of these patients temporarily required total parenteral nutrition in that regard. Moreover, the author has seen a substantial number of superb weight loss results in extremely heavy (BMI > 70 kg/m^2) patients after distal RYGB. Patients in this weight class frequently experience poor weight loss after short-limb RYGB [9,13].

In summary, the risk/benefit analysis of distal/malabsorptive RYGB is complex. A well-controlled prospective comparative study of short limb versus distal/malabsorptive RYGB would require years to complete. It would be extremely helpful for the insurance carriers to enjoin bariatric surgeons in conduct of such a study. It seems that the National Institute of Health has no interest in supporting such a study because they dropped the surgical arm of the Study of Health Outcomes of Weight-loss Trial (and changed its name) in 2000.

Revisional bariatric operations

The long-term "success rate" of conventional short-limb RYGB ranges between 50% and 80%, which implies "failure" for the remaining patients [3,9,13,17]. Weight loss "failure" is significantly more prevalent in superobese patients (BMI ≥ 50 kg/m^2). Fortunately, surgical options are available for patients who fail to achieve satisfactory loss after short-limb RYGB. Adding restriction alone to a failed RYGB rarely results in substantial weight loss [18–20]. Conversely, adding malabsorption by lengthening the Roux limb has provided good long-term weight loss for many of these challenging patients. In Sugerman et al's [8] report, the 22 patients who failed conventional RYGB lost an additional 30% of their excess weight with improvement or resolution of the comorbidities that reoccurred with cessation of weight loss following conventional RYGB. Likewise, Fobi et al [21] reported substantial additional weight loss after conversion of patients who failed conventional banded RYGB to a more malabsorptive procedure, again at the expense of more metabolic complications. The author has performed 29 distal RYGBs with up to a 75-cm common channel in patients who had unsatisfactory weight loss after conventional RYGB, including 10 who had a 150-cm Roux limb. Mean weight loss was 32.5 kg at 1 year postconversion. Twenty of the 29 patients (72.4%) lost at least 50% of their excess weight. Metabolic sequelae and diarrhea accompanied these revisions. One patient required takedown of her RYGB because of poor weight loss in conjunction with severe hypocalcemia and hypoproteinemia. Noncompliant, unreliable patients with poor weight loss after conventional RYGB should not be offered revisional surgery;

however, preoperative identification of these noncompliant patients is problematic.

Summary

RYGB that is performed with at least a 150-cm Roux limb results in significantly greater weight loss than shorter (<100-cm) Roux limb procedures in superobese patients (BMI $\geq$ 50 kg/m^2). Conversely, longer Roux limb procedures do not provide greater weight loss in less obese (BMI < 50 kg/m^2) patients. Modest elongation of the Roux limb—in the range of 150 cm to 200 cm—does not result in more frequent nutritional sequelae compared with shorter Roux limb procedures. Conversely, RYGBs, in which the Roux or the biliopancreatic limb is very long with anastomosis to the mid or distal ileum (very, very long), usually results in more metabolic problems than RYGBs in which the Roux limb measures up to 150 cm and the biliopancreatic limb is short. The current (2005) CPT codes do not stratify Roux limb length adequately on the basis of weight loss outcome or late nutritional sequelae.

References

[1] Lechner GW, Callender K. Subtotal gastric exclusion and gastric partitioning: a randomized prospective comparison of one hundred patients. Surgery 1981;90:637–44.
[2] Pories WJ, Flickinger EG, Meelheim D, et al. The effectiveness of gastric bypass over gastric partition in morbid obesity. Consequence of distal gastric and duodenal exclusion. Ann Surg 1982;196:389–99.
[3] Yale CE. Gastric surgery for morbid obesity: Complications and long term weight control. Arch Surg 1989;124:941–7.
[4] Measurement of overweight. Stat Bull NY Metropol Life Insur Co 1984;54:20–3.
[5] Brolin RE, Kenler HA, Gorman JG, et al. Long-limb gastric bypass in the superobese: a prospective randomized study. Ann Surg 1992;215:387–95.
[6] Bruder SJ, Freeman JB, Brazeau-Gravelle P. Lengthening the Roux-Y limb increases weight loss after gastric bypass: a preliminary report. Obes Surg 1991;7:414–9.
[7] Freeman JB, Kotlarewsky M, Phoenix C. Weight loss after extended gastric bypass. Obes Surg 1997;7:337–44.
[8] Sugerman JH, Kellum JM, DeMaria EJ. Conversion of proximal to distal gastric bypass for failed gastric bypass for superobesity. J Gastrointest Surg 1997;1:517–25.
[9] MacLean LD, Rhode BM, Nohr CW. Late outcome of isolated gastric bypass. Ann Surg 2000;231:524–8.
[10] MacLean LD, Rhode BM, Nohr CW. Long or short-limb gastric bypass? J Gastrointest Surg 2001;5:525–30.
[11] Choban PS, Flancbaum LJ. The effect of Roux limb lengths on outcome after Roux-en-Y gastric bypass: a prospective randomized clinical trial. Obes Surg 2002;12:540–5.
[12] Feng JJ, Gagner M, Pomp A, et al. Effect of standard vs. extended Roux limb length on weight loss outcomes after laparoscopic Roux-en-Y gastric bypass. Surg Endosc 2003;17: 1055–60.

[13] Brolin RE, Lamarca LB, Kenler HA, et al. Malabsorptive gastric bypass in patients with superobesity. J Gastrointest Surg 2002;6:195–205.

[14] Murr MM, Balsiger BM, Kennedy FP, et al. Malabsorptive procedures for severe obesity: comparison of pancreaticobiliary bypass and very, very long Roux-en-Y gastric bypass. J Gastrointest Surg 1998;3:607–12.

[15] Current Procedure Terminology CPT 2004. Chicago: AMA Press; 2004.

[16] Fischer JE. Serving on the MAP of the Blue Cross and Blue Shield Association's TEC. Bull Am Coll Surg 2004;89:22–5.

[17] Halverson JD, Zuckerman GR, Koehler RE, et al. Gastric bypass for morbid obesity: a medical-surgical assessment. Ann Surg 1981;194:152–60.

[18] Sugerman HJ, Wolper JL. Failed gastroplasty for morbid obesity. Am J Surg 1984;148: 331–6.

[19] Behrns KE, Smith CD, Kelly KA, et al. Reoperative bariatric surgery: lessons learned to improve patient selection and results. Ann Surg 1993;218:646–53.

[20] Naslund I. The size of the gastric outlet and the outcome of surgery for obesity. Acta Chir Scand 1986;152:205–10.

[21] Fobi M, Lee H, Igwe D Jr, et al. Revision of failed gastric bypass to distal Roux-en-Y gastric bypass; a review of 65 cases. Obes Surg 2001;11:190–5.

ELSEVIER
SAUNDERS

SURGICAL
CLINICS OF
NORTH AMERICA

Surg Clin N Am 85 (2005) 819–833

The Duodenal Switch Operation for Morbid Obesity

Gary J. Anthone, MD, FACS

Morbid obesity is defined as having a body mass index (BMI) of greater than 40 kg/m² or being 100 pounds over ideal body weight as defined by the 1983 Metropolitan Life Insurance tables [1]. Although environmental factors clearly are important, identical twin studies [2] and ongoing elucidation of the functional roles of hormones, such as leptin [3,4] and ghrelin [5], have shown that genetic and physiologic factors have a major role in the etiology of this disease. In the United States, morbid obesity has reached epidemic proportions. Two percent of men and 6% of women—a total of approximately 12 million Americans—are morbidly obese. The disease is associated with an increased risk of serious comorbidities, including type II diabetes, sleep apnea, cardiovascular diseases, and orthopedic disabilities. It recently was estimated that individuals who have morbid obesity have a mortality risk similar to that of smokers [6]. A 25-year-old man with a BMI of 45 kg/m² can expect to lose approximately 14 years of life [7].

Nonoperative treatments for patients who have morbid obesity have not been shown to produce reliable long-term benefit; consequently, surgical therapy has become the preferred treatment [8]. It is estimated that 98,000 surgical procedures were performed in 2003, compared with 63,000 in 2002, and 47,000 in 2001 [9]. The 1991 National Institutes of Health consensus conference on morbid obesity recommended that surgery be considered for well-informed patients who have acceptable operative risks [10]. Although the intention of the conference was not to recommend or condemn a particular surgical procedure, two surgical procedures—the vertical banded gastroplasty and Roux-en-Y gastric bypass—were discussed as surgical alternatives. The biliopancreatic diversion, gastric banding, and duodenal switch procedures were not discussed at this conference but have gained popularity over

Bariatric Surgery Program, Physicians Clinic, Nebraska Methodist Health System, 10060 Regency Circle, Omaha, NE 68114, USA.

E-mail address: ganthon@nmhs.org

0039-6109/05/$ - see front matter © 2005 Elsevier Inc. All rights reserved.
doi:10.1016/j.suc.2005.03.007   surgical.theclinics.com

the past several years for a variety of reasons, whereas the vertical banded gastroplasty has become less popular.

The jejunoileal bypass in 1953 was the first surgical procedure that was designed to produce weight loss [11]. The severe hepatic, metabolic, and nutritional complications of this procedure [12] led to the development of the loop gastric bypass [13]; the vertical banded gastroplasty [14]; and eventually, the currently performed Roux-en-Y gastric bypass [15]. In 1979, Scopinaro et al [16] described the biliopancreatic diversion procedure that combined a subtotal distal gastrectomy with a long limb Roux-en-Y and 50-cm common channel reconstruction to induce fat malabsorption specifically.

The duodenal switch procedure was described by DeMeester et al [17] in 1987 as a surgical solution for primary bile reflux gastritis or to decrease the postgastrectomy symptoms that are seen in patients after distal gastrectomy and gastroduodenostomy. Later that year, Hess adapted this procedure to the treatment of morbid obesity by adding a 75% longitudinal gastrectomy to reduce gastric capacity and acid production and extending the Roux limb to a length similar to that recommended by Scopinaro to induce fat malabsorption (Fig. 1) [18]. The rationale for the longitudinal gastrectomy was to preserve the pylorus and first portion of the duodenum which negates the possibility of dumping symptoms and decrease the risk of marginal ulcers.

Despite favorable reports on the use of the duodenal switch procedure for the treatment of morbid obesity [18–24], it has been slow to gain widespread

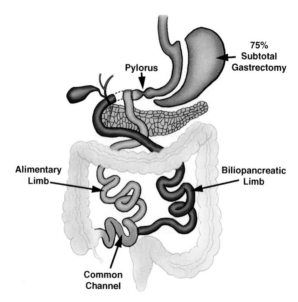

Fig. 1. The duodenal switch procedure performed for the treatment of morbid obesity. The operation consists of a 75% longitudinal gastrectomy, creation of an alimentary limb that is approximately 50% of total small bowel length, and a common channel length of 100 cm. A cholecystectomy is performed routinely.

popularity. There are three reasons for this: (1) there is a perception that its malabsorptive component may be associated with metabolic complications, protein calorie malnutrition, or other nutrient deficiencies; (2) the procedure is longer and more technically demanding than other bariatric operations; and (3) the procedure is difficult to perform laparoscopically. Many surgeons and patients believe that the duodenal switch offers many advantages in the short- and long-term over that of the Roux-en-Y gastric bypass or gastric banding procedures. Patients should be informed about the various surgical procedures for weight loss before making a decision to have surgery.

Operative technique

The surgery is performed by way of an upper midline incision using the Gomez retractor (Pilling Surgical, Horsham, Pennsylvania; Fig. 2). The triangular ligament of the left lateral liver segment is incised to expose the area of the hiatus. After ligating all gastroepiploic and short gastric vessels, a 75% longitudinal gastrectomy is performed, leaving a tubularized stomach of approximately 100 cm^3 (Fig. 3). The duodenum is divided proximal to the ampulla, about 4 cm beyond the pylorus at the level of the gastroduodenal artery. The small bowel length is measured and divided at its midpoint; the distal end (alimentary limb) is brought through a window that is created in the transverse mesocolon and anastomosed to the proximal duodenum (Fig. 4). The proximal end of the divided small bowel, now the distal end of the biliopancreatic limb, is anastomosed to the ileum 100 cm from the ileocecal valve to create a 100-cm common channel (see Fig. 1). A cholecystectomy is performed at the same time because of the high incidence of gallstone formation after this type of procedure. A Jackson-Pratt drain and feeding jejunostomy are placed before closure of the abdomen (Fig. 5). On postoperative day 2 or 3, a video swallow is performed to exclude extravasation of contrast or anastomotic stenosis; if normal, a clear liquid

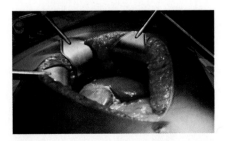

Fig. 2. Midline incision with placement of the Gomez retractor system. Note the large size of the liver which makes exposure of the hiatus difficult whether open or laparoscopic surgery is performed.

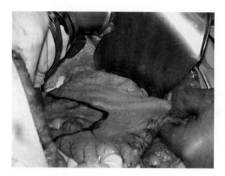

Fig. 3. The longitudinal gastrectomy is performed by resecting along a line parallel to, and approximately 2 cm from, the lesser curvature. This produces a tubularized stomach of approximately 100 cm³.

diet is started. Most patients are taking a solid diet at the time of their discharge on the fourth or fifth postoperative day.

Postoperatively, as is standard after most bariatric procedures, patients are followed initially at 3 and 6 weeks, at then every 3 months during the first year, every 6 months during the second year, and yearly thereafter. A complete blood count, chemical metabolic profiles, and parathyroid hormone levels are obtained at each visit starting 3 months postoperatively. Patients are instructed repeatedly to take daily vitamin and mineral supplementation.

Results

The results of the duodenal switch procedure have been reproduced by several investigators with similar outcomes [18–24]. The largest and most current series was reported by the author when working at the University of Southern California and is used to illustrate these results.

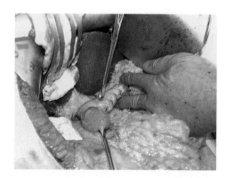

Fig. 4. Air insufflation of the retrocolic duodenoenterostomy anastomosis. Note the lack of tension at the suture line.

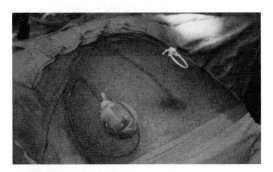

Fig. 5. Jackson-Pratt drain on right and feeding jejunostomy tube on left. Skin is closed using a subcuticular technique.

Demographic details

The demographic data for a total of 701 patients who underwent the duodenal switch procedure for weight loss, and for men and women separately, are shown in Table 1. The preoperative weight, excess body weight (EBW), and BMI were significantly greater in men. Fifty-eight percent of the patients (407) were supermorbidly obese, with a BMI that was at least 50 kg/m^2. Twenty-two percent of the patients (155) had a preoperative BMI that was at least 60 kg/m^2. The propensity for a higher incidence of men having surgery and for supermorbidly obese patients is typical for most open series of weight loss procedures compared with other laparoscopic series. Accrual of patients increased progressively over the 10-year period; most patients (66%) were operated on during the last 3 years (Fig. 6).

Weight loss

Fig. 7 shows the mean and 95% confidence intervals for percentage of EBW loss (%EBWL) for all patients at 6, 12, 36, and at least 60 months after surgery. Table 2 shows the mean and median for weight loss, %EBWL, and BMI for the total study population. Patient weight and BMI were

Table 1
Demographic data for the total and female and male patients. Continuous data are shown as mean (S.D.)

	Total patients	Female	Male	P value
Number of patients	701 (100%)	549 (78.3%)	152 (21.7%)	–
Age (y)	42.3 (10.4)	41.9 (10.3)	43.5 (10.7)	.1
Weight (lb)	331.2 (73.4)	314.9 (57.7)	390.4 (91.7)	<.001
Excess body weight (lb)	191.3 (66.9)	180.3 (55.3)	231.1 (87.2)	<.001
BMI (kg/m^2)	52.3 (9.6)	52.1 (8.9)	55.1 (11.3)	<.001

P values are for the comparison of men versus women and were calculated using Student *t* test.

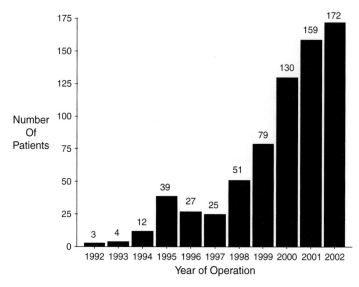

Fig. 6. Yearly accrual rate of patients who had a duodenal switch procedure as their primary weight loss operation during the period of the study. The number of patients per year is shown above the bar.

significantly lower, and the %EBWL was significantly higher, at all postoperative intervals compared with the preoperative values.

The %EBWL for men and women was similar (Fig. 8). Patients with a preoperative BMI of at least 50 kg/m^2 had a slightly lower %EBWL at all postoperative intervals compared with patients with a preoperative BMI of

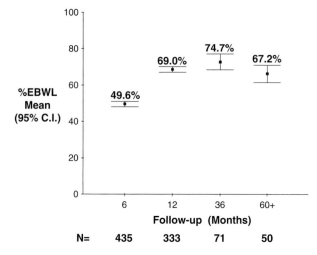

Fig. 7. Percent excess body weight loss (%EBWL) for all patients. Graph shows mean and 95% confidence intervals (C.I.) for the mean.

Table 2
Postoperative weight loss for the total study population

Follow-up interval	6 months	12 months	36 months	≥ 60 months
Number of patients	435	333	71	50
Weight lost (lb)				
Mean (S.D.)	89.2 (25.9)	126.9 (40.6)	131.4 (49.5)	117.9 (45.9)
Median	86	122	120	103
EBWL (%)				
Mean (S.D.)	49.6 (15.5)	68.7 (14.2)	72.8 (18.5)	66.3 (16.7)
Median	48.3	69.0	74.7	67.2
BMI (kg/m^2)				
Mean (S.D.)	38.4 (7.3)	32.4 (6.2)	31.1 (6.7)	32.5 (6.8)
Median	37.3	31.7	29.7	30.7

less than 50 kg/m^2; however, this difference was not statistically significant after the first postoperative year (Fig. 9). Table 3 shows the mean weight loss, the BMI, and the %EBWL for patients with a preoperative BMI of less than 50 kg/m^2 and at least 50 kg/m^2. The success rate of the procedure, using the criterion of the loss of at least 50% of EBW for the total patients and those with a preoperative BMI of less than and at least 50 kg/m^2, is shown in Fig. 10. Even in superobese patients (preoperative BMI $\geq$ 50 kg/m^2), the success rate was 78.6% and 73.3% at 3 and 5 or more years, respectively.

Nutritional and metabolic parameters, dietary volume, and bowel function

Maximum weight loss occurred by 3 years after operation and represents the time of maximal metabolic and nutritional challenge. At this time

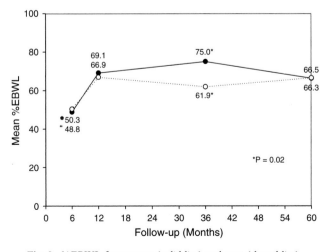

Fig. 8. %EBWL for women (*solid line*) and men (*dotted line*).

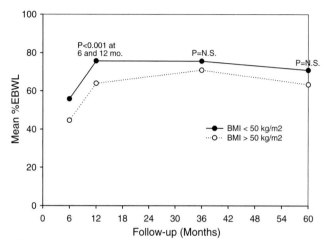

Fig. 9. %EBWL and preoperative BMI. N.S., not significant.

interval, the percentage of patients who had normal serum values was
98.3% for albumin (normal range 3.2–5.0 g/dL); 70.7% for total calcium
(normal range 8.5–10.3 mg/dL); and 51.7% for hemoglobin (normal range:
13.8–17.2 g/dL [men] and 12.0–15.6 g/dL [women]; Table 4). With the
exception of 40 patients who required readjustment of the length of the

Table 3
Weight loss in patients with a preoperative BMI < 50 kg/m^2 and BMI ≥ 50 kg/m^2

Follow-up interval	6 months	12 months	36 months	≥60 months
Preoperative BMI < 50 kg/m^2				
N	173	134	29	20
Weight loss (lb)				
Mean (S.D.)	75.2 (16.1)	102.4 (22.3)	104.4 (24.7)	91.9 (27.5)
Median	75	102	105	90.5
%EBWL (%)				
Mean (S.D.)	55.8 (10.8)	75.7 (14.3)	75.6 (15.2)	70.9 (15.3)
Median	55.4	75	75.2	70.4
BMI (kg/m^2)				
Mean (S.D.)	32.1 (3.7)	27.7 (3.4)	27.7 (3.7)	28.3 (3.7)
Median	31.7	27.7	27.7	28.2
Preoperative BMI ≥ 50 kg/m^2				
N	262	199	42	30
Weight loss (lb)				
Mean (S.D.)	98.5 (27.1)	143.4 (41.8)	149.9 (53.9)	135.3 (47.7)
Median	97	137	141	139
%EBWL (%)				
Mean (S.D.)	44.6 (8.7)	63.9 (11.9)	70.9 (20.4)	63.3 (17.1)
Median	44.9	63.9	70.9	65.8
BMI (kg/m^2)				
Mean (S.D.)	42.6 (6.2)	35.6 (5.7)	33.5 (7.3)	35.4 (6.9)
Median	41.4	34.8	32.8	34.2

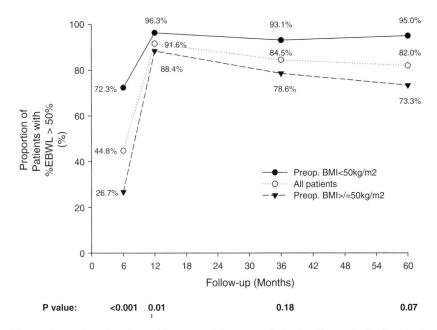

Fig. 10. Proportion of patients with a successful outcome, defined as %EBWL of at least 50%. *P* values for the comparison of the super morbidly obese patients (BMI > 50 kg/m²) with the morbidly obese patients (BMI < 50 kg/m²) are shown at the bottom of the graph at the specific follow-up intervals (Fisher's exact test).

common channel, no clinical sequelae have occurred from hypocalcemia or anemia. Of importance, there was no clinical evidence of hepatic dysfunction.

Table 5 shows (1) the patients' assessment of ingested volume as a percentage of their preoperative volume, (2) the dietician's estimate of daily caloric intake, and (3) the mean number of bowel movements per day. Despite a gradual increase in dietary volume and caloric intake, weight loss was maintained; this indicates that the malabsorptive component of the procedure is effective. The observation that the mean caloric intake was limited to less than 1700 calories per day indicates that the restrictive component also was working. These benefits were achieved with minimal to no restrictions on the types of food ingested. Bowel habits were altered minimally, despite a 100-cm common channel. Dumping did not occur, which indicated that in addition to preservation of the pylorus, vagal control of gastrointestinal function was maintained.

Morbidity and mortality

Perioperative (in-hospital and 30-day postoperative) deaths occurred in 10 of the 701 (1.4%) patients. The causes of death were pulmonary embolus in 4 patients, rhabdomyolysis in 2 patients, and duodenal stump leak, gastric

Table 4
Serum nutritional and metabolic measures. Data are shown as mean (S.D.)

Follow-up interval	Preoperative	6 months	12 months	36 months
Serum albumin				
Number of patients	646	339	255	58
Serum albumin (g/dL)	4.1 (0.3)	3.9 (0.5)	3.9 (0.5)	4.1 (0.4)
Within normal range (3.2–5.0 g/dL) (%)	99.7%	93.5%	94.1%	98.3%
Serum hemoglobin				
Number of patients	658	343	256	60
Serum hemoglobin (g/dL)	13.6 (1.2)	13.0 (1.2)	12.5 (1.3)	11.9 (1.6)
Within normal range (%) (Female: > 12.0 g/dL) (Male: > 13.8 g/dL)	88.6%	75.8%	63.7%	51.7%
Serum calcium				
Number of patients	660	340	256	58
Serum calcium	9.2 (0.6)	9.0 (0.5)	8.9 (0.5)	8.6 (0.6)
Within normal range (8.5–10.5 mg/dL) (%)	96.2%	89.1%	79.3%	70.7%

leak, cecal necrosis, and aspiration pneumonia in 1 patient each. Demographic data for the 10 patients who died are shown in Table 6. Male gender, older age, and higher preoperative BMI were associated significantly with perioperative mortality.

Significant perioperative morbidity occurred in 21 patients (2.9%). Nonfatal leaks occurred at the duodenoenteric anastomosis in 1 patient, at the enteroenterostomy anastomosis in 1 patient, at the duodenal stump in

Table 5
Dietary intake and bowel frequency

Follow-up interval	Preoperative	6 months	12 months	36 months	≥ 60 months
Volume of food ingested (% of preoperative amount)					
Number of patients	–	418	315	63	47
Mean (S.D.)	–	41.7 (14.8)	52.6 (16.6)	62.9 (19.5)	62.7 (18.8)
Median	–	40	50	50	65
Caloric intake (calories/d)					
Number of patients	–	258	194	30	–
Mean (S.D.)	–	1137.5 (486.9)	1363.6 (537.6)	1642.5 (710.9)	–
Median	–	1095	1297	1582	–
Bowel frequency (Number of bowel movements/d)					
Number of patients	43	421	316	65	48
Mean (S.D.)	1.9 (0.9)	2.7 (1.6)	2.6 (1.5)	2.8 (2.2)	2.8 (1.8)
Median	2.0	2.5	2.0	2.0	2.5

Table 6
Demographic factors associated with perioperative mortality. Continuous variable data are as shown as median (range)

	Perioperative mortality	No perioperative mortality	P value
Male:female	6:4	146:545	0.009*
Age at operation(y)	51 (33–65)	42 (16–71)	0.01**
Body mass index (kg/m^2)	63.5 (47–76)	51 (34–95)	0.004**

 * P value calculated using Fisher's exact test.
 ** P value calculated using Mann-Whitney test.

1 patient, and at the gastric staple line in 2 patients. Splenectomy to control bleeding was necessary in 3 patients. Four patients required postoperative exploratory laparotomy: 2 for bleeding, 1 for small bowel obstruction, and 1 for presumed abdominal sepsis. Four out of 6 patients recovered from gluteal rhabdomyolysis. Wound dehiscence occurred in 5 patients.

Revisional surgery to increase the length of the common channel was necessary in 40 patients (5.7%). Reoperation was driven by evidence of malnutrition as reflected by hypoalbuminemia, peripheral edema, or continued weight loss (34 patients); persistent diarrhea, despite a restriction of fat intake and medication use (4 patients); or chronic unexplained abdominal pain (2 patients).

Discussion

The published reports of the duodenal switch prove that it is a safe and effective primary operation for the treatment of morbid obesity. The safety of the procedure is evident by the operative mortality of 1% to 2%, which is comparable to that of other large weight loss surgical series [25,26]. Similar to other series, male gender, older age, and superobesity are significant risk factors for mortality. Other studies of open and laparoscopic bariatric surgery have reported lower mortality rates; however, these series included a lower proportion of men and superobese patients. The morbidity of the duodenal switch procedure also is similar to that of reports on the open gastric bypass procedure [25,26]. Of note is the fact that the anastomotic leak rate of the duodenal switch is low compared with the Roux-en-Y gastric bypass. This likely is due to the close proximity of the bowel, and thus, the lack of tension on the duodenoenteric anastomosis compared with the gastroenteric anastomosis that is performed near the cardia in the standard gastric bypass procedure. The risk of leakage from the longer longitudinal gastric suture line is minimal and is comparable to the leak rate from the gastric staple line in the gastric bypass procedure.

The duodenal switch operation includes a restrictive and a malabsorptive component. This has resulted in conflicting opinions regarding the side effects of the malabsorptive component; some investigators believe that severe metabolic and nutritional complications are frequent after the operation. This likely is due to a presumed similarity of the currently performed malabsorptive operations (ie, biliopancreatic diversion and duodenal switch) to the old and now-discredited jejunoileal bypass. Unlike the jejunoileal bypass, the duodenal switch does not have a blind enteric limb. Rather, both limbs are stimulated, one with food and the other with biliopancreatic secretions; this prevents mucosal atrophy, bacterial over-growth, and liver injury. Instances of liver failure after the duodenal switch operation do not seem to be different from that of other gastric bypass operations, and most likely are a result of pre-existing liver disease. The results of the duodenal switch procedure on liver histology—by studying biopsy specimens before and after weight loss—demonstrate that lobular inflammation or necrosis, fatty change, and a portal fibrosis score were decreased or unchanged in most patients [27].

Modification of the Roux-en-Y gastric bypass—by lengthening the Roux limb and shorting the common channel—has been proposed for patients who have more extreme degrees of obesity or when the routine Roux-en-Y bypass has failed. This "long-limb" or distal gastric bypass has been associated with significant metabolic and nutritional complications that have been assumed inappropriately to occur with the duodenal switch procedure [28–30]. The hypoalbuminemia and other nutritional deficits that are observed in patients who undergo a long-limb gastric bypass may be secondary to the combination of extreme gastric restriction—which is imposed by the small gastric pouch—and a malabsorptive component. In contrast, the duodenal switch procedure allows patients to ingest approxi-mately two thirds of their preoperative dietary volume without specific food intolerances; more than 98% maintain a serum albumin within the normal range 3 years after surgery.

A certain percentage of patients develop anemia and hypocalcemia after any operation which bypasses the duodenum, including Roux-en-Y gastric bypass and the duodenal switch. This is because iron and calcium are absorbed preferentially in the distal duodenum and proximal jejunum. The frequency of anemia after duodenal switch ($\sim 50\%$) is comparable to that reported by Brolin et al [30] after Roux-en-Y gastric bypass, where it varied from 41% after a short limb to 74% after a long Roux limb. After the duodenal switch procedure, the degree of anemia usually is mild; however, in a small percentage of patients it proves refractory to oral iron sup-plementation, although a portion of duodenum remains. These patients do, however respond to parenteral iron injections. Vitamin B12 deficiencies do not occur in patients after the duodenal switch in contrast to the 35% incidence that was reported after Roux-en-Y gastric bypass [30]. This likely is due to the preservation of more gastric mucosa with the duodenal switch procedure. Reports of studies of the duodenal switch operation on calcium and parathyroid hormone metabolism have demonstrated that patients do not develop clinical evidence of hypocalcemia or bone loss [31].

The magnitude of weight loss that occurs after the duodenal switch procedure is better than that achieved after the Roux-en-Y gastric bypass procedure. Although criteria for satisfactory weight loss are not well-defined in the literature, loss of 50% of EBWL is accepted broadly as a measure of success. In the study by MacLean et al [32] on isolated gastric bypass, only 57% of patients who had supermorbid obesity (BMI > 50 kg/m^2) achieved this goal. In contrast, 73% of patients with a BMI of at least 50 kg/m^2 achieved success by this criterion at 5 or more years after duodenal switch operation in our study; even greater success rates were reported by Hess and Hess [18].

If the mortality and morbidity of the duodenal switch are comparable to other common weight loss procedures, what advantage does it have to offset the longer operative time and technical difficulty? Most investigators and patients believe that the answer relates to quality of life. Although it is unquestioned that morbidly obese patients must adopt some behavioral change of their eating habits, bariatric procedures that use a small proximal gastric pouch and Roux-en-Y limb are characterized by a much more extreme restriction of intake and the development of a higher rate of marginal ulcerations and dumping syndrome. It is stated commonly that the dumping symptoms that follow carbohydrate-rich foods act as a deterrent to eating, and are an integral component of the mechanism of action of the Roux-en-Y gastric bypass. After the duodenal switch procedure, patients can consume a wide variety of foods, and can ingest a volume that is approximately half of their preoperative intake, without the fear of dumping. This permits restoration of social functioning and good quality of life.

Summary

The duodenal switch provides excellent weight loss with preservation of good alimentation, even in the superobese. This is accomplished with acceptable operative mortality and minimal dietary limitations and metabolic sequelae. The results of the duodenal switch that are reported in the literature should remove any inhibitions that exist about the use of this procedure as treatment for patients who have morbid obesity.

References

[1] Anthone GJ. Surgery for morbid obesity. In: Zuidema GD, Yeo CJ, editors. Shackelford's surgery of the alimentary tract. Philadelphia: W.B. Saunders; 2002. p. 437–47.

[2] Stunkard AJ, Harris JR, Pedersen NL, et al. The body-mass index of twins who have been reared apart. N Engl J Med 1990;322:1483–7.

[3] Zhang Y, Proenca R, Maffei M, et al. Positional cloning of the mouse obese gene and its human homologue. Nature 1994;372:425–32.

[4] Friedman JM. Obesity in the new millennium. Nature 2000;404:632–4.

[5] Cummings DE, Weigle DS, Frayo RS, et al. Plasma ghrelin levels after diet-induced weight loss or gastric bypass surgery. N Engl J Med 2002;346:1623–30.

[6] Peeters A, Barendregt JJ, Willekens F, et al. NEDCOM The Netherlands Epidemiology and Demography Compression of Morbidity Research Group. Obesity in adulthood and its consequences for life expectancy: a life-table analysis. Ann Intern Med 2003;138:24–32.

[7] Fontaine KR, Redden DT, Wang C, et al. Years of life lost due to obesity. JAMA 2003;289: 187–93.

[8] Patterson EJ, Urbach DR, Swanstrom LL. A comparison of diet and exercise therapy versus laparoscopic Roux-en-Y gastric bypass surgery for morbid obesity: a decision analysis model. J Am Coll Surg 2003;196:379–84.

[9] Mitka M. Surgery for obesity: demand soars amid scientific, ethical questions. JAMA 2003; 289:1761–2.

[10] NIH Consensus Development Conference Draft Statement on Gastrointestinal Surgery for Severe Obesity. Obes Surg 1991;257–65.

[11] Kremen AJ, Linner JH, Nelson C. An experimental evaluation of the nutritional importance of proximal and distal small intestine. Ann Surg 1954;140:439–44.

[12] DeWind LT, Payne JH. Intestinal bypass surgery for morbid obesity. Long-term results. JAMA 1976;236:2298–301.

[13] Mason EE, Ito C. Gastric bypass. Ann Surg 1969;170:329–39.

[14] Printen KJ, Mason EE. Gastric surgery for relief of morbid obesity. Arch Surg 1973;106: 428–31.

[15] Griffin WO, Young VL, Stevenson CC. A prospective comparison of gastric and jejunoileal bypass procedures for morbid obesity. Ann Surg 1977;186:500–9.

[16] Scopinaro N, Gianetta E, Civalleri D, et al. Bilio-pancreatic bypass for obesity: II. Initial experience in man. Br J Surg 1979;66:618–20.

[17] DeMeester TR, Fuchs KH, Ball CS, et al. Experimental and clinical results with proximal end-to-end duodenojejunostomy for pathologic duodenogastric reflux. Ann Surg 1987;206: 414–26.

[18] Hess DS, Hess DW. Biliopancreatic diversion with a duodenal switch. Obes Surg 1998;8: 267–82.

[19] Lagace M, Marceau P, Marceau S, et al. Biliopancreatic diversion with a new type of gastrectomy: some previous conclusions revisited. Obes Surg 1995;5:411–8.

[20] Marceau P, Biron S, Bourque RA, et al. Biliopancreatic diversion with a new type of gastrectomy. Obes Surg 1993;3:29–35.

[21] Marceau P, Hould FS, Simard S, et al. Biliopancreatic diversion with duodenal switch. World J Surg 1998;22:947–54.

[22] Baltasar A, Bou R, Bengochea M, et al. Duodenal switch: an effective therapy for morbid obesity–intermediate results. Obes Surg 2001;11:54–8.

[23] Rabkin RA. Distal gastric bypass/duodenal switch procedure, Roux-en-Y gastric bypass and biliopancreatic diversion in a community practice. Obes Surg 1998;8:53–9.

[24] Anthone GJ, Lord RV, DeMeester TR, et al. The duodenal switch operation for the treatment of morbid obesity. Ann Surg 2003;238:618–28.

[25] Pories WJ, Swanson MS, MacDonald KG, et al. Who would have thought it? An operation proves to be the most effective therapy for adult-onset diabetes mellitus. Ann Surg 1995;222: 339–50.

[26] Livingston EH, Huerta S, Arthur D, et al. Male gender is a predictor of morbidity and age a predictor of mortality for patients undergoing gastric bypass surgery. Ann Surg 2002;236: 576–82.

[27] Abramyan L, Kanel G, Anthone GJ, et al. Severity of nonalcoholic fatty liver disease (NAFLD) after surgical weight loss in patients with morbid obesity [abstract]. Gastroenterology 2003;124:A825.

[28] Sugerman HJ, Kellum JH, DeMaria EJ. Conversion of proximal to distal gastric bypass for failed gastric bypass for superobesity. J Gastrointest Surg 1997;1:517–24.

[29] Murr MM, Balsiger BM, Kennedy FP, et al. Malabsorptive procedures for severe obesity: comparison of pancreaticobiliary bypass and very very long limb Roux-en-Y gastric bypass. J Gastrointest Surg 1999;3:607–12.

[30] Brolin RE, LaMarca LB, Kenler HA, et al. Malabsorptive gastric bypass in patients with superobesity. J Gastrointest Surg 2002;6:195–203.

[31] Marceau P, Biron S, Lebel S, et al. Does bone change after biliopancreatic diversion? J Gastrointest Surg 2002;6:690–8.

[32] MacLean LD, Rhode BM, Nohr CW. Late outcome of isolated gastric bypass. Ann Surg 2000;231:524–8.

ELSEVIER
SAUNDERS

SURGICAL
CLINICS OF
NORTH AMERICA

Surg Clin N Am 85 (2005) 835–852

Bariatric Surgical Outcomes

Mohamed R. Ali, MD*, William D. Fuller, MD,
Michael P. Choi, DO, Bruce M. Wolfe, MD

*Department of Surgery, University of California, Davis Medical Center, 2221 Stockton
Boulevard, Cypress Building, Sacramento, CA 95817, USA*

In Western society, morbid obesity has become an increasingly costly public health issue, in terms of the serious medical illnesses that are associated with this condition and the number of dollars that are spent on treatment. Currently, the number of overweight individuals in the world is estimated at 1.7 billion [1]. In the United States, the problem is at epidemic proportions. It has been estimated that up to two thirds of the population of the United States is overweight, and that half of these individuals can be classified as obese [1]. The spread of obesity has been well-documented since 1980, with significant increases occurring in the adolescent population and in individuals who are 18 to 29 years old [2–4]. Currently, 15 million individuals in the United States can be characterized as morbidly obese (Body Mass Index [BMI] > 35 kg/m^2) [5]. The condition seems to be particularly prevalent in populations with the least access to medical care, such as ethnic minorities, as well as in poorly-educated and impoverished populations; this stresses the potential for huge burdens on the health care system from this treatable condition [6].

Morbid obesity

As a result of the severity of obesity as a medical problem, the National Institutes of Health convened in 1985 and again in 1991. From these consensus conferences, criteria for treating morbid obesity were developed, including medical and surgical solutions. Furthermore, the 1991 consensus conference deemed surgery as the best method for achieving weight loss, maintaining long-term weight loss, and effectively addressing the serious comorbidities that are associated with obesity. Roux-en-Y gastric bypass

---
* Corresponding author.
E-mail address: mohamed.ali@ucdmc.ucdavis.edu (M.R. Ali).

0039-6109/05/$ - see front matter © 2005 Elsevier Inc. All rights reserved.
doi:10.1016/j.suc.2005.03.005   *surgical.theclinics.com*

(RYGB) and vertical banded gastroplasty (VBG) were identified as the best surgical procedures for accomplishing sustained weight loss and addressing medical comorbidities [7]. Since then, the Surgeon General of the United States has characterized morbid obesity as a disease that is treated most effectively with bariatric surgery.

Surgery as treatment for morbid obesity

It is believed that the first surgery to attempt to correct obesity was performed by Dr. Richard Varco at the University of Minnesota in 1953 [5]. This first attempt at weight loss surgery, the jejunoileal bypass, has since been abandoned because of the numerous complications that stemmed from the high degree of malabsorption that resulted in malnutrition, severe diarrhea, and neurologic complications.

Since that time, the field of bariatric surgery has evolved into several types of procedures to produce weight loss. Broadly, bariatric surgical procedures can be grouped based on the mechanism through which it is believed that weight loss is achieved: (1) procedures that act largely through malabsorption (biliopancreatic diversion [BPD] with or without duo-denal switch [DS]), (2) procedures that act largely through restriction (VBG, adjustable gastric banding), and (3) procedures that act through a combination of malabsorption and restriction (RYGB). Some of these procedures—unique in the mechanism of weight loss, the number of com-plications, and the long-term success—have been subjected to scrutiny through randomized trials; however, most have been studied mainly through retrospective reviews and cohort studies.

This article attempts to describe the procedures that are performed for weight loss and characterize the associated short-term success (operative safety, in-hospital morbidity/mortality) and long-term efficacy (weight loss, weight loss maintenance, postoperative complications). It discusses each category of procedure and reviews the current outcomes literature. It also addresses the technical challenges that are involved with the performance of each procedure and how these challenges may affect short and long-term outcomes. It concludes by comparatively analyzing the outcomes of the various bariatric surgical procedures and their respective roles in effectively managing the morbidly obese patient.

Malabsorptive procedures

Techniques

The malabsorptive surgical model to achieve weight loss largely was practiced in the 1950s. Interest in malabsorptive procedures waned with the realization of associated complications. This interest was resurrected in the

1970s and 1980s with the evolution from the earlier jejunoileal bypass to the BPD to the current variation, the BPD with DS (BPD/DS).

The BPD achieves weight loss primarily through malabsorption as a result of increased gastric emptying rates and accelerated intestinal transit times [8]. The technique of BPD, as originally conceived, included a partial gastrectomy with closure of the duodenal stump. The small intestine was divided at the midpoint between the ligament of Treitz and the ileocecal valve to create a Roux-en-Y gastroenterostomy. The enteroileostomy was positioned to create a 50-cm common channel to the ileocecal valve [9].

Subsequent modifications of the procedure included changes in how the gastrectomy is performed, the length of small bowel used for the common channel, anastomotic techniques, and the addition of other surgical procedures that are designed to decrease gastric volume and to reduce complications of malabsorption while maintaining high degrees of long-term weight loss. These adaptations have been used with some success by surgeons, and the results have been reported with follow-up of patients up to 20 years in some instances.

A popular variation on the technique of BPD is the addition of the "DS." As originally proposed for BPD by Hess, a vertical sleeve gastrectomy was constructed, and division of the duodenum was performed just distal to the pylorus. This allowed normal filling of the gastric remnant and maintenance of physiologic sensation of satiety. Also, the sleeve gastrectomy added an element of restriction to the procedure while reducing parietal cell mass in the fundus. In theory, this would reduce the incidence of marginal ulceration [10]. This technique also has been adapted to a laparoscopic approach that was popularized by a group of surgeons led by Gagner [11,12].

Complications

Scopinaro et al [8] published a 20-year experience with the BPD. Several nutrition-related abnormalities that are associated with this procedure have been identified. Calcium deficiency may be profound and lead to bone demineralization. Anemia—secondary to reduced absorption of iron and decreased activity of gastric intrinsic factor—has been documented. Thiamine deficiency that led to neurologic complications has been shown. Notably, protein enteropathies have been associated with the procedure; however, with adequate supplementation, these phenomena may be minimized. Postoperative supplementation with calcium, iron, folate, thiamine, vitamin B12, and fat soluble vitamins usually is necessary.

The phenomenon of protein malnutrition has been dealt with in several ways by investigators who perform the BPD. There is a recognized relationship between gastric volume and severity of protein enteropathy. Larger gastric volumes have been associated with slower transit times and greater protein absorption; however, constructing larger gastric reservoirs comes at the cost of reduced weight loss. Attempts at altering the length of the alimentary limb to increase nutrient absorption resulted in a decreased incidence of protein malnutrition [8].

Results of trials using BPD with or without DS have been reported in several large series (Table 1) [9]. Mortality rates have been low, ranging from 0% to 1.9%. The most prevalent surgical complications include incisional hernia (18%) and anastomotic ulcer (6.3%–10.6%). Similar complication rates were demonstrated when the laparoscopic approach was compared with the open approach (Table 2) [13]. A retrospective comparative study by Kim et al [13] in 2003 reported a 2-year experience with 54 superobese patients who underwent laparoscopic or open BPD/DS. The investigators concluded that morbidity and mortality were similar between patients who underwent the two procedures. They noted that morbidity and mortality

Table 1

Complications following biliopancreatic diversion and duodenal switch

Complication	1998 Scopinaro BPD (N = 1356)	1998 Marceau BPD (N = 252)	1999 Totte BPD (N = 180)	1998 Marceau BPD/DS (N = 465)
Operative mortality	9 (0.7%)	4 (1.6%)	0	9 (1.9%)
Anastomotic leak	–	1	–	4
Pancreatitis	–	2	–	–
Pulmonary embolus	4	1	–	3
Sleep apnea	–	–	–	1
Malignant hyperthermia	1	–	–	1
Cardiac arrest	3	–	–	–
Wound infection	1	–	–	–
Postoperative morbidity	38 (2.8%)	42 (16.7%)	29 (16.1%)	76 (16.3%)
Gastric performation	1 (0.07%)	–	–	–
Gastric retention	–	23 (9.1%)	11 (6.1%)	29 (6.2%)
Duodenal blowout	–	–	2 (1.1%)	–
Anastomotic fistula	2 (0.1%)	2 (0.8%)	1 (0.6%)	8 (1.7%)
Pancreatitis	–	2 (0.8%)	1 (0.6%)	8 (1.7%)
Intraperitoneal bleed	3 (0.2%)	–	–	–
Abdominal abscess	–	–	–	–
Wound infection	13 (1.0%)	2 (0.8%)	9 (5.0%)	5 (1.0%)
Wound dehiscence	9 (0.7%)	–	–	–
Deep thrombophlebitis	4 (0.3%)	–	2 (1.1%)	–
Acute psychosis	–	–	1 (0.6%)	–
Others	–	5 (2.0%)	–	9 (1.9%)
Late complications	–	–	32 (17.8%)	–
Incisional hernia	–	–	32 (17.8%)	–
Intestinal occlusion	–	–	2 (1.1%)	–
Anastomotic ulcer	86 (6.3%)	–	19 (10.6%)	–
Protein malnutrition	91 (6.7%)	–	2 (1.1%)	–
Hemorrhoids	79 (5.8%)	–	–	–

From Van Hee R. Biliopancreatic diversion in the surgical treatment of morbid obesity. World J Surg 2004;28:438; with permission.

Table 2
Comparison of clinical data and preoperative comorbid conditions in patients undergoing laparoscopic and open BPD-DS

Results	Laparoscopic BPD/DS	Open BPD/DS	P value
Median opt time (min)	210 ± 68	259 ± 60	NS
Median est blood loss (ml)	100 ± 130	300 ± 285	NS
Median length of stay (d)	4 ± 41	5 ± 47	NS
Comorbidity (% of patients)			
Hypertension	57.6	42.8	
Arthritis	26.9	28.5	
Asthma	19.2	21.4	
Diabetes	26.9	32.1	
Sleep apnea	46.1	46.4	
Major complications			
Subphrenic abscess	1	0	
Anastomotic leak	1	0	
Respiratory failure	1	1	
Wound disruption	0	0	
Incisional hernia	1	0	
Urinary tract infection	0	1	
Total complications	6 (23%)	5 (17%)	
Mortality	2 (7.6%)	1 (3.5%)	

Abbreviations: est, estimated; NS, not significant; opt, operative.

Adapted from Kim WW, Gagner M, Kini S, et al. Laparoscopic vs. open biliopancreatic diversion with duodenal switch: a comparative study. J Gastrointest Surg 2003;7(4):554,555; with permission.

were greater than in the typical obese population that underwent gastric bypass surgery but that patients in the study population were superobese individuals in whom the rate of complications would tend to be higher, even with gastric bypass. The laparoscopic group also attained acceptable weight loss that ranged up to 76 kg at 1 year [13]. Reduced wound complications (wound infections and incisional hernias), reduced abdominal wall trauma, and better exposure of the gastroesophageal region for the surgeon are some of the advantages of the laparoscopic approach. Although the laparoscopic approach is feasible and seems comparable with the open technique, longer follow-up and randomized studies are necessary to demonstrate this clearly.

Weight loss

The BPD/DS has been demonstrated to provide excellent excess body weight loss (EBWL). In their early experience with BPD/DS, Hess and Hess [10] evaluated 440 patients. With follow-up approaching 8 years, they noted 70% EBWL in superobese patients (BMI > 50 kg/m^2). Maximum weight loss was noted at 2 years postoperatively (80% EBWL). In another study, EBWL was 74% ± 15% at 2-year follow-up [8].

In a comparative study of more than 14,964 patients who underwent bariatric surgery, weight loss reported with BPD/DS was among the highest values attained in bariatric surgery (Table 3) [9]. BPD/DS has been shown to provide profound and sustained weight loss in the superobese patient [11]. Similar levels of weight loss can be achieved with open or laparoscopic BPD/DS (Table 4) [12,13].

Improvement in comorbidities

Patients who undergo BPD/DS show significant improvement in comorbid conditions after surgery. A study of 54 superobese patients who underwent BPD/DS demonstrated a 71% improvement in diabetes and a 20% improvement in hypertension [13].

A recent meta-analysis that was undertaken by Buchwald et al [1] corroborates improvement in comorbidities postoperatively in patients who undergo BPD/DS. In diabetic patients who underwent BPD/DS, 98.9% had complete resolution of diabetes. Similarly, 83% of hypertensive patients had resolution of hypertension after surgery. Other conditions that demonstrated improvement included obstructive sleep apnea (71.2%), hyperlipidemia (99.9%), and hypertriglyceridemia (100.0%) [1].

Conclusion

Few clinical trials have examined the role of BPD/DS in bariatric surgery. From existing data, it is evident that the superobese patient can achieve excellent weight loss. With BPD/DS, these patients need to be monitored intensively for potential nutritional and metabolic abnormalities and receive aggressive prophylactic supplementation. The procedure can be performed safely, and its outcomes, weight loss, and effects on comorbid conditions are comparable with, or in some instances, superior to, other bariatric procedures. Although the technical learning curve may be steep with laparoscopic BPD/DS, it can be performed safely with excellent results [8].

Table 3
Comparative overview of weight loss in 54 studies, performed in 14,964 patients according to the bariatric operation

Operative procedure	Total patients	% EBW (loss)	% BMI (loss)
Gastric banding	4429	48.6	22.2
Biliopancreatic diversion	3903	68.8	35.5
Vertical banded gastroplasty	3382	58.3	29.0
Roux-en-Y gastric bypass	2949	68.6	34.7
Long-limb RYGB	301	71.6	33.9

Abbreviation: EBW, excess body weight.
From Van Hee R. Biliopancreatic diversion in the surgical treatment of morbid obesity. World J Surg 2004;28:440; with permission.

Table 4
Excess body weight loss after laparoscopic (Lap) and open BPD-DS

Characteristics	Lap BPD/DS	Open BPD/DS	P value
3-mo weight loss (kg)	35.6 ± 15.6	32.2 ± 14.7	NS
6-mo weight loss (kg)	56.9 ± 20.4	44.3 ± 5.7	NS
9-mo weight loss (kg)	68.1 ± 26.5	48.7 ± 4.1	NS
12-mo weight loss	76.7 ± 19.7	56.8 ± 26.3	NS
> 12-mo change in BMI	37.3 ± 5.6	48.2 ± 6.3	NS

From Kim WW, Gagner M, Kini S, et al. Laparoscopic vs. open biliopancreatic diversion with duodenal switch: a comparative study. J Gastrointest Surg 2003;7(4):556; with permission.

Malabsorptive/restrictive

Techniques

Gastric bypass was first performed by Mason and Ito in 1966 [14]. In this variation, a horizontal distal gastrectomy was performed to create a gastric reservoir to which a loop of jejunum was anastomosed. Revisions, including a decrease in the volume of the gastric pouch, leaving the excluded stomach in situ, draining the pouch by way of a Roux-en-Y jejunal limb, and the introduction of the laparoscopic technique, have been among the major advances in the procedure [5].

Current variations in the surgical technique include the method by which the gastric pouch is created, the technique of gastrojejunostomy, and the configuration and length of the alimentary and biliopancreatic limbs. With the increase in the performance of laparoscopic gastric bypass, first popularized by Wittgrove and Clark, the effect of these alterations on outcomes has been studied extensively [15–18]. This section reviews the experience with RYGB and discusses recent outcomes of the laparoscopic technique.

Complications

Several large series have reported outcomes of RYGB. These were reviewed in a recent analysis which examined more than 3000 cases from 17 different studies (Tables 5 and 6) [18]. Wound complications (incisional hernias and wound infections) are prevalent within these studies of open gastric bypass procedures. Anastomotic leak (1.68%) and pulmonary embolus (0.78%), although infrequent, were reported consistently.

The open and laparoscopic techniques have shown equality in terms of safety. Procedurally, variations in the technique of gastrojejunostomy, passage of the Roux limb (antecolic/retrocolic), and positioning of the gastrojejunostomy (antegastric/retrogastric) have been reported [15–17]. In a review of a 20-year experience with 3000 open and laparoscopic RYGB procedures, the incidence of anastomotic leak was 2.3% in the open group and 4.2% in the laparoscopic group [19]. Kellum et al [20] reported a 1.2%

Table 5
Complications in selected series of open gastric bypass

	Oh, et al (1997)	Fobi, et al (1998)	Kirkpatrick (1998)	MacLean, et al (2000)	Balsiger, et al (2000)	Nguyen, et al (2001)	Livingston, et al (2002)	Total
Patients (n)	194	705	212	274	191	76	1067	2719
PE	NA	4/705	3/212	1/274	1/191	1/76	9/1067	19/2525
Leak	0/194	9/705	13/212	NA	1/191	2/76	15/1067	40/2445
Bowel obstruction	1/194	28/705	NA	6/274	8/191	0/76	10/1067	53/2507
GI bleed	NA	NA	NA	NA	1/191	0/76	7/1067	8/1334
Wound infection	2/194	NA	NA	NA	11/191	8/76	NA	21/461
Stomal stenosis	6/194	4/705	NA	NA	2/191	2/76	1/1067	15/2233
Ventral hernia	16/194	32/705	NA	40/274	32/191	6/76	NA	126/1440
Splenic injury	0/194	3/705	NA	NA	1/191	0/76	NA	4/1166
Pneumonia	1/194	NA	NA	NA	3/191	NA	0/1067	4/1452
Death	0/194	3/705	4/212	1/274	1/191	0/76	14/1067	23/2719

Abbreviations: GI, qastrointestinal; PE, pulmonary embolus.
Data from Podnos Y, Jimenez J, Wilson S, et al. Complications after laparoscopic gastric bypass: a review of 3464 cases. Arch Surg 2003;138:959.

Table 6
Complications in selected series of laparoscopic gastric bypass

Study (year)	n	PE	Leak	Bowel obstruction	GI bleed	Wound infections	Stomal stenosis	Ventral hernia	Pneumonia	Death
Schauer, et al (2000)	275	2/275	12/275	3/275	3/275	24/275	13/275	2/275	1/275	1/275
Wittgrove, et al (2000)	500	NA	11/500	3/500	NA	28/500	8/500	0/500	NA	0/500
Nguyen, et al (2001)	79	0/79	1/79	3/79	3/79	1/79	9/79	0/79	NA	0/79
Higa, et al (2001)	1500	3/1500	14/1500	52/1500	NA	2/1500	73/1500	4/1500	1/1500	3/1500
Dresel, et al (2002)	100	0/100	3/100	5/100	3/100	2/100	3/100	1/100	NA	0/100
DeMaria, et al (2002)	281	3/281	14/281	5/281	NA	3/281	18/281	5/281	NA	0/281
Papasavas, et al (2002)	116	1/116	3/116	12/116	2/116	NA	4/116	NA	NA	1/116
Oliak, et al (2002)	300	2/300	4/300	5/300	NA	20/300	6/300	NA	1/300	3/300
Gould, et al (2002)	223	NA	4/223	4/223	NA	17/223	12/223	2/223	NA	0/223
Total	3374	11/2651	66/3374	92/3374	11/570	97/3258	146/3374	14/2958	3/2075	8/3374

Data from Podnos Y, Jimenez J, Wilson S. Complications after laparoscopic gastric bypass: a review of 3464 cases. Arch Surg 2003;138:959.

incidence of anasomotic leak. Other studies documented leak rates as low as 0.1% [17]. Using a totally hand-sewn approach for the gastrojejunostomy, Higa et al [21] have performed a large number of surgeries without an anastomotic leak. These studies also suggest that the rate of anastomotic leaks decreases with the level of experience of the surgeon and that a steep learning curve contributes to leak rates.

Pulmonary embolism, one of the more devastating complications in bariatric surgery, remains a potentially mortal event. The application of the laparoscopic approach to bariatric surgery has added the potential theoretic increase in the incidence of thromboembolic events perioperatively. Patients are placed in reverse Trendelenburg position for long periods of time, and pneumoperitoneum may impede venous return. Despite the use of pharmaceutical and mechanical prophylaxis, pulmonary embolism is reported as a complication of bariatric surgery with a similar incidence in laparoscopic and open techniques [21–23].

The application of minimally invasive surgery to gastric bypass has led to studies that compared the open approach with the laparoscopic approach. Nguyen et al [22] reviewed complications by comparing prospective data from patients who underwent laparoscopic RYGB with retrospective data on patients who underwent open gastric bypass (Table 7). Similar rates of morbidity were noted between the two approaches, including leaks and pulmonary emboli. Incisional hernia rates in the open group were significantly greater than in the laparoscopic group. In a more recent prospective, randomized trial between the two approaches, similar findings were reported. Lujan et al [23] found similar rates of early complications

Table 7
Perioperative complications in patients undergoing laparoscopic and open gastric bypass

Complications	Lap RYGB	Open RYGB	P value
Major complications			
Intra-op hemorrhage	0	2	
Gastrointestinal bleed	1	1	
Anastamotic leak	0	1	
Bowel obstruction	1	0	
Respiratory failure	1	1	
Severe wound infection	0	2	
Pulmonary embolism	0	0	
DVT	0	0	
Total (%)	3 (8.6%)	7 (20%)	NS
Minor complications			
Ileus	1	0	
Minor wound infection	1	1	
Urinary tract infection	0	1	
Total (%)	2 (5.7%)	2 (5.7%)	NS

Abbreviations: DVT, deep vein thrombosis; Intra-op, intraoperative.
From Nguyen N, Ho H, Palmer L, et al. A comparison study of laparoscopic versus open gastric bypass for morbid obesity. J Am Coll Surg 2000;191(2):153; with permission.

(22.6% versus 29.4%) between the laparoscopic and open approaches. Late complications, made up mainly of incisional hernias were more numerous in the open group (11% versus 24%). The incidence of marginal ulcer and anastomotic stricture was reported to be greater with the laparoscopic technique [19]. Also, early and late bowel obstructions seem to have a greater incidence with the laparoscopic approach [22].

The significant learning curve for performing laparoscopic gastric bypass has been implicated in increased rates of some complications, such as anastomotic leaks, wound infections, and bowel obstruction secondary to internal hernia [24,25]. Surgical techniques have evolved to address some of the challenges of laparoscopic gastric bypass. Precise closure of all defects (mesenteric defects and Petersen defect), although not advocated by some investigators [26], has been demonstrated clearly to decrease the incidence of small bowel obstruction secondary to internal hernia [27,28]. Passage of the Roux limb in an antecolic position also may avoid narrowing that might occur at the defect in the transverse mesocolon during the retrocolic approach [27].

Weight loss

Weight loss following gastric bypass surgery has been studied extensively. Mean EBWL after open RYGB ranges from 57% to 65% at 1 year [30]. Similar EBWL has been reported with laparoscopic RYGB. In one of the first reports of the outcomes of laparoscopic gastric bypass, Schauer et al [25] found that EBWL following laparoscopic RYGB was 68% at 1 year and 83% at 2 years. Other studies have corroborated these findings [23,29,30,31].

Improvement in comorbidities

With the recognition of the metabolic syndrome (combination of hypertension, dyslipidemia, glucose intolerance, and obesity), morbidly obese patients have been identified as being at high risk for this condition. If left untreated, the progression to cardiovascular disease has been documented in these patients. Weight loss is critical to the treatment of this condition. One year postoperatively, metabolic syndrome can be reversed in up to 98% of patients [32].

Much has been written about the medical conditions that are associated with morbid obesity and their response to gastric bypass surgery. Diabetes, hypertension, hypercholesterolemia, and obstructive sleep apnea are the among the commonly reported comorbid conditions which tend to improve significantly or resolve completely following RYGB [6,15,23,31–33]. Pories et al [34] reported a 14-year experience with more than 600 patients; 98.7% of subjects who had glucose intolerance and 82.9% who had noninsulin-dependent diabetes mellitus developed a normal serum level of glucose and glycosylated hemoglobin within 1 year postoperatively. In a recent review of a 5-year experience with 1160 patients, Schauer et al [33] identified complete resolution of type 2 diabetes mellitus in 83% of diabetic patients following laparoscopic RYGB. This study also demonstrated that patients with a long history of diabetes and those who required insulin were less likely to experience complete resolution of the disease; however, these patients still exhibited significant improvement in their conditions.

Hypertension also seems to respond favorably to gastric bypass. In a study of 1000 patients, Sugerman et al [32] reported that 60% to 73% of hypertensive individuals enjoyed complete resolution of their disease. African American patients tended to experience a diminished response; only 60% experienced resolution of hypertension following surgery.

A meta-analysis of more than 136 studies, totaling more than 22,000 patients, recently was undertaken by Buchwald et al [1]. Diabetes mellitus and glucose intolerance demonstrated concomitant improvement in hemoglobin A1C levels and fasting glucose in 83% of affected patients. Hypertension resolved completely in 67.5% of affected patients and improved in up to 87%. Similarly, hyperlipidemia (96.9% improvement), obstructive sleep apnea (94.8% resolution or improvement), gastroesophageal reflux disease, pseudo-tumor cerebri, urinary stress incontinence, and other comorbid conditions demonstrated variable, but positive, response to RYGB.

Compelling data also have been gathered regarding the improvement in quality of life that is experienced by patients who have undergone RYGB [35,36]. Although the success of bariatric surgery often is measured in terms of EBWL and improvement in medical comorbidities, the psychosocial response of the patient deserves important consideration. Several instruments that focus on health-related quality of life have been used to attempt to quantify this subjective measure. It is apparent that reduction in weight or improvement in comorbidities does not correlate necessarily with improved quality of life.

The laparoscopic approach has demonstrated a more rapid improvement in quality of life than the open approach. In a comparison of patients who underwent laparoscopic and open RYGB at 6 months postoperatively, 97% of patients who underwent laparoscopic gastric bypass reported good or better quality of life by bariatric analysis and reporting outcome system compared with only 82% in the open group [35]. Additionally, patients who underwent the laparoscopic procedure returned to work and normal daily activity sooner and had a shorter hospitalization than patients who underwent open gastric bypass.

Conclusions

RYGB usually is considered to be the standard bariatric surgical procedure. Excellent sustained weight loss and profound improvement in medical comorbidities can dramatically alter the lives of patients. In its laparoscopic iteration, RYGB is a procedure that requires advanced training and is associated with a significant learning curve. Although its principal mode of functioning is through its restrictive component, hormonal changes that accompany gastric bypass may contribute to weight loss. Even as laparoscopy has helped to reduce some of the morbidity that is associated with gastric bypass, it remains a serious operation that requires technical expertise to optimize surgical outcomes.

Restrictive procedures

Techniques

Mason and Printen performed the first restrictive procedure for weight loss in 1971 [5]. They performed a horizontal gastroplasty using the greater curvature of the stomach as the outlet. Early variations on the gastroplasty did not accomplish adequate weight loss. Patients circumvented the reduced gastric outlet by altering their dietary habits, and sweet-eaters were able to gain weight. Subsequent modifications to this procedure led to the development of the VBG, in which a vertical gastric pouch is created along the lesser curvature, and a band is used to restrict the gastric outlet [5].

The adjustable gastric band (AGB) was developed by Kuzmak [37] and further refined with the adoption of laparoscopy [38,39]. By percutaneously injecting saline into a subcutaneous port, the size of the outlet can be adjusted. The AGB often is considered to be the least invasive of bariatric surgical procedures because the gastrointestinal tract is not disrupted, anastomosed, or anatomically reconfigured. A small pouch and stoma are created by placing a band around the upper portion of the stomach. Laparoscopic placement of the gastric band is associated with reduced pain and faster recovery. Additionally, AGB allows for adjustment in the postoperative period, which can assist the surgeon and the patient in calibrating the gastric outlet for desired weight loss without the need for further surgery. Banding procedures are largely reversible, and this often is cited as an advantage.

Complications

Long-term data on complications that are associated with gastric banding are not available in the United States. In Europe and Australia, where the experiences have been more extensive, more long-term data are available. Many of the complications of gastric banding seem to be associated with the learning curve, which may be significant, even in the hands of the advanced laparoscopic surgeon [40]. Early complications that are associated with laparoscopic AGB include wound and port-site infections, band slippage, and gastric perforation [42,43]. Band slippage was reported to occur in 21% to 36% of cases [41–43]. This complication frequently required reoperation. Refinements in the techniques of band placement reduced the incidence of band slippage, decreased the rate of reoperation, and improved weight loss. These include the pars flaccida dissection as opposed to the epigastric approach [44].

Band erosion was reported to occur in 0.2% to 2% of cases [41,42]. A variety of factors has been hypothesized to cause band erosion, including an overly tightened band, inadvertently suturing the band to the stomach, and local infection. Leakages from the subcutaneous port and band tubing have been described. Gastric perforation, not identified at the time of surgery, also has been reported [45]. Additionally, some patients (29%) developed esophagitis without band slippage.

A recent prospective randomized trial compared the results of AGB with VBG [46]. This study demonstrated that early morbidity was greater for VBG than AGB (9.8% versus 6.1%), whereas AGB had more numerous complications than VBG (32.7% versus 9.8%). Several reoperations were performed in patients who had AGB, mainly because of severe esophagitis, reflux disease, band slippage, and poor dietary compliance.

VBG compares favorably with the RYGB in terms of complication rates. Lower morbidity and less nutritional difficulties were reported for VBG when compared with RYGB [47].

Weight loss

Restrictive bariatric procedures do not achieve EBWL that is equivalent to the malabsorptive or mixed procedures. Patients who undergo VBG may demonstrate 47% EBWL at 2 years postoperatively [46]. Longer-term EBWL was reported at 44% with 10 years of follow-up [47]. In a prospective, randomized trial, weight loss following VBG was inferior to weight loss following RYGB, particularly in African American patients and sweet-eaters [48].

It has been hypothesized that these differences may be due to the inability of the VBG to restrict the intake of high-calorie liquids and the ability of the pouch to expand with overeating. Many patients take advantage of these phenomena to circumvent the procedure. The VBG has not been successful for individuals who report a lifestyle of eating sugars and simple carbohydrates. For these individuals, the gastric bypass may be the preferred procedure [48].

AGB does not achieve weight loss similar to VBG (39% EBWL at 1 year for AGB versus 62.3% EBWL for VBG) [46]. DeMaria [41] reported similar EBWL at 3 years (38%) with AGB. Patients who were sweet-eaters, diabetic, or African American exhibited poor weight loss with AGB. Meta-analysis of 1848 patients showed an EBWL of 47.5% in banded patients [1].

Improvement in comorbidities

Data seem to suggest that diabetes, hypertension, dyslipidemia, and obstructive sleep apnea respond positively to AGB. A recent meta-analysis demonstrated resolution of these conditions in 47.9%, 43.2%, 58.9%, and 95% of affected patients, respectively [1]. Longer-term studies from Europe demonstrated marked improvement in diabetes mellitus (86%), hypertension (75%), hyperlipidemia (95%), and pulmonary disorders (95%) after 6 years of follow-up [49].

Although data exist on the long-term effects of VBG on weight loss, less information is available regarding its effects on medical comorbidities. The resolution of diabetes (71.6%), hypertension (69.9%), dyslipidemia (73.6%), and obstructive sleep apnea (78.2%) following VBG is less than that reported for RYGB [1].

Conclusions

Restrictive procedures achieve weight loss through reduction of intake by reducing the size of the gastric reservoir and restricting the outlet. Gastrointestinal continuity essentially is preserved.

Several technical challenges account for the learning curve of these procedures. As a class, restrictive procedures generally are safe, but late complications are plentiful and may require reoperation.

Weight loss and improvement in associated medical conditions is inferior to other classes of bariatric procedures. Certain patient behaviors may compromise the amount of weight that is lost after restrictive bariatric operations; however, banding procedures and gastroplasty techniques may be valuable in properly-selected patients.

Summary

Morbid obesity is a disease that is treated most successfully with surgery. The armamentarium with which the surgeon may approach this disease has increased in diversity and complexity since the initial distal intestinal bypasses that were performed in the last century. As our understanding of the etiology of obesity has improved, the procedures have been adapted to treat this disease better.

The approach to each bariatric patient should be individualized. Although weight loss and improvement in health are paramount goals of obesity surgery, the manner in which these goals are attained need not be driven completely by dogma and mystery. Using evidence-based trials, bariatric surgical procedures have been refined, and continue to undergo further development. Through this outcomes-driven approach, bariatric procedures have become increasingly safe and efficacious.

Choosing the appropriate procedure for each patient should not be based solely on a menu-driven approach. Although weight loss by BPD tends to be the most profound and this operation may be suited better to the superobese patient; this has not been demonstrated definitively. For individuals who are at risk for nutritional problems and in whom the irreversibility of RYGB is unacceptable, a banding procedure may be preferred. A sweet-eater will fail a banding procedure and may be more likely to succeed with a gastric bypass. The safety and efficacy of all of these procedures have been demonstrated. Clearly, steep learning curves exist for all; however, by using an intelligent and sound approach to preoperative work-up, meticulous surgical technique, prompt response to complications, and sustained postoperative follow-up, favorable outcomes can be achieved.

References

[1] Buchwald H, Avidor Y, Braunwald E, et al. Bariatric surgery: a systematic review and meta-analysis. JAMA 2004;292(14):1724–37.

[2] Mokdad A, Serdula M, Dietz W, et al. The spread of the obesity epidemic in the United States, 1991–1998. JAMA 1999;282(16):1519–22.

[3] Flegal K, Carroll M, Ogden C, et al. Prevalence and trends in obesity among US adults, 1999–2000. JAMA 2002;288(14):1723–7.

[4] Hedley A, Ogden C, Johnson C, et al. Prevalence of overweight and obesity among US children, adolescents, and adults, 1999–2002. JAMA 2004;291(23):2847–50.

[5] Buchwald H, Buchwald J. Evolution of operative procedures for the management of morbid obesity 1950–2000. Obes Surg 2002;12:705–17.

[6] Livingston E, Ko C. Socioeconomic characteristics of the population eligible for obesity surgery. Surgery 2004;135(3):288–96.

[7] Livingston E. Obesity and its surgical management. Am J Surg 2002;184:103–13.

[8] Scopinaro N, Adami G, Marinari G, et al. Biliopancreatic diversion. World J Surg 1998;22: 936–46.

[9] Van Hee HGG. Biliopancreatic diversion in the surgical treatment of morbid obesity. World J Surg 2004;28:435–44.

[10] Hess D, Hess D. Biliopancreatic diversion with a duodenal switch. Obes Surg 1998;8:267–82.

[11] Feng J, Gagner M. Laparoscopic biliopancreatic diversion with duodenal switch. Semin Laparosc Surg 2002;9(2):125–9.

[12] Ren C, Patterson E, Gagner M. Early results of laparoscopic biliopancreatic diversion with duiodenal switch: a case series of 40 consecutive patients. Obes Surg 2000;10(6):514–23.

[13] Woo-Woo K, Gagner M, Kini S, et al. Laparoscopic vs. open biliopancreatic diversion with duodenal switch: a comparative study. J Gastrointest Surg 2003;7(4):552–7.

[14] Mason EE, Ito C. Gastric bypass in obesity, 1967. Obes Res 1996;4(3):316–9.

[15] Wittgrove A, Clark G. Laparoscopic gastric bypass, Roux en-Y 500 patients: technique and results, with 3–60 month follow-up. Obes Surg 2000;10:233–9.

[16] Abdel-Galil E, Sabry A. Laparoscopic Roux-en-Y gastric bypass-evaluation of three different techniques. Obes Surg 2002;12:639–42.

[17] Carrasquilla C, English W, Esposito P, et al. Total stapled, total intra-abdominal laparoscopic Roux-en-Y gastric bypass: one leak in 1,000 cases. Obes Surg 2004;14:613–7.

[18] Podnos Y, Jimenez J, Wilson S, et al. Complications after laparoscopic gastric bypass: a review of 3464 cases. Arch Surg 2003;138:957–61.

[19] Fernandez A, DeMaria E, Tichansky D, et al. Experience with over 3,000 open and laparoscopic bariatric procedures: multivariate analysis of factors related to leak and resultant mortality. Surg Endosc 2004;18:193–7.

[20] Kellum J, DeMaria E, Sugerman H. The surgical treatment of morbid obesity. Curr Probl Surg 1998;35:791–858.

[21] Higa K, Boone K, Ho T. Complications of the laparoscopic Roux-en-Y gastric bypass: 1,040 patients-what have we learned? Obes Surg 2000;10:509–13.

[22] Nguyen N, Ho H, Palmer L, et al. A comparison study of laparoscopic versus open gastric bypass for morbid obesity. J Am Coll Surg 2000;191(2):149–55.

[23] Lujan J, Frutos D, Hernandez Q, et al. Laparoscopic versus open gastric bypass in the treatment of morbid obesity: a randomized prospective study. Ann Surg 2004;4(239): 433–7.

[24] Schauer P, Ikramuddin S, Gourash W, et al. Outcomes after laparoscopic roux-en-y gastric bypass for morbid obesity. Ann Surg 2000;232(4):515–29.

[25] Schauer P, Ikramuddin S, Hamad G, et al. The learning curve for laparoscopic Roux-en-Y gastric bypass is 100 cases. Surg Endosc 2003;17:212–5.

[26] Champion J, Williams M. Small bowel obstruction and internal hernias after laparoscopic Roux-en-Y gastric bypass. Obes Surg 2003;13:596–600.

[27] Felsher J, Brodsky J, Brody F. Small bowel obstruction after laparoscopic Roux-en-Y gastric bypass. Surgery 2003;134(3):501–5.

[28] Higa K, Ho T, Boone K. Internal hernias after laparoscopic Roux-en-Y gastric bypass: incidence, treatment and prevention. Obes Surg 2003;13:350–4.

[29] DeMaria E, Sugerman H, Kellum J, et al. Results of 281 consecutive total laparoscopic Roux-en-Y gastric bypasses to treat morbid obesity. Ann Surg 2002;2325(5):640–7.

[30] Perugini R, Mason R, Czerniach D, et al. Predictors of complication and suboptimal weight loss after laparoscopic Roux-en-Y gastric bypass: a series of 188 patients. Arch Surg 2003; 138:541–6.

[31] Lee W, Huang M, Wang W, et al. Effects of obesity surgery on the metabolic syndrome. Arch Surg 2004;139:1088–92.

[32] Sugerman H, Wolfe L, Sica D, et al. Diabetes and hypertension in severe obesity and effects of gastric bypass-induced weight loss. Ann Surg 2003;237(6):751–8.

[33] Schauer P, Burguera B, Ikramuddin S, et al. Effect of laparoscopic Roux-en Y gastric bypass on type 2 diabetes mellitus. Ann Surg 2003;238(4):467–85.

[34] Pories W, Swanson M, MacDonald K, et al. Who would have thought it? An operation proves to be the most effective therapy for adult-onset diabetes mellitus. Ann Surg 1995; 222(3):339–50.

[35] Ballantyne G. Measuring outcomes following bariatric surgery: weight loss parameters, improvement in co-morbid conditions, change in quality of life and patient satisfaction. Obes Surg 2003;13:954–64.

[36] Nguyen N, Goldman C, Rosenquist J, et al. Laparoscopic versus open gastric bypass: a randomized study of outcomes, quality of life, and costs. Ann Surg 2001;234(3): 279–91.

[37] Kuzmak L. Silicone gastric banding: a simple and effective operation for morbid obesity. Contemp Surg 1986;28:13–8.

[38] Broadbent R, Tracy M, Harrington P. Laparoscopic gastric banding: a preliminary report. Obes Surg 1993;3:63–7.

[39] Catona A, Gossenberg M, La Manna A, et al. Laparoscopic gastric banding: preliminary series. Obes Surg 1993;3:207–9.

[40] Shapiro K, Patel S, Abdo Z, et al. Laparoscopic adjustable gastric banding. Surg Endosc 2004;18:48–50.

[41] DeMaria E. Laparoscopic adjustable silicone gastric-banding: complications. J Laparoendosc Adv Surg Tech A 2003;13(4):271–7.

[42] Weber M, Muller M, Bucher T, et al. Laparoscopic gastric bypass is superior to laparoscopic gastric banding for treatment of morbid obesity. Ann Surg 2004;240(6):975–83.

[43] Martikainen T, Pirenen E, Alhava E, et al. Long-term results, late complications and quality of life in a series of adjustable gastric banding. Obes Surg 2004;14:648–54.

[44] Ren C, Fielding G. Laparoscopic adjustable gastric banding: surgical technique. J Laparoendosc Adv Surg Tech A 2003;13(4):257–63.

[45] Ren C, Weiner M, Allen J. Favorable early results of gastric banding for morbid obesity. Surg Endosc 2004;18:543–6.

852 ALI et al

[46] Morino M, Toppino M, Bonnet G, et al. Laparoscopic adjustable silicone gastric banding versus vertical banded gastroplasty in morbidly obese patients: a prospective randomized controlled clinical trial. Ann Surg 2003;238(6):835–42.

[47] Fobi M. Vertical banded gastroplasty vs gastric bypass: 10 years follow-up. Obes Surg 1993; 3:161–4.

[48] Sugerman H, Londrey G, Kellum J, et al. Weight loss with vertical banded gastroplasty and Roux-en-Y gastric bypass for morbid obesity with selective versus random assignment. Am J Surg 1989;57(1):93–102.

[49] Mittermair R, Weiss H, Nehoda H, et al. Laparoscopic Swedish Adjustable Gastric Banding: 6-year follow-up and comparison to other laparoscopic bariatric procedures. Obes Surg 2003;13:412–7.

SURGICAL
CLINICS OF
NORTH AMERICA

Surg Clin N Am 85 (2005) 853–868

Complications of Bariatric Surgery

Edward H. Livingston, MD, FACS[a,b]

[a]*Division of Gastrointestinal and Endocrine Surgery,
University of Texas Southwestern School of Medicine,
5323 Harry Hines Boulevard, Room E7-126, Dallas, TX 75390-9156, USA*
[b]*Veterans Administration, North Texas Health Care System,
4500 South Lancaster Road, Dallas, Texas 75216, USA*

The rise in bariatric operations has been exponential, with a greater acceptance for these procedures [1,2]. Although complication rates are relatively low (major complications occur in approximately 10% of procedures), they can result in formidable disability [1,3–6]. Adverse outcomes also result in medical malpractice claims that are particularly problematic for bariatric surgery practices. For these reasons, surgeons performing these operations must be knowledgeable and must possess the technical skills required for managing complications when they occur. The purpose of this article is to review the major complications that occur following anti-obesity procedures and to provide recommendations regarding their management.

In general, bariatric surgery patients have little physiologic reserve and, because of their large size, do not manifest complications in the same manner as normal-sized patients. For example, obese patients with peritonitis may not have fevers, abdominal pain or tenderness, or an elevated white blood cell count that one would expect when intrabdominal sepsis is present. Obese patients may only have tachycardia in the face of significant intrabdominal pathology. Of all the manifestations of intrabdominal sepsis, tachycardia with a pulse exceeding 120 beats per minute is the most consistent and reliable physical finding [7]. For this reason, when postoperative bariatric surgery patients become this tachycardic, the clinicians caring for them should assume that an intrabdominal abscess or anastomotic leak is present. Imaging studies in these patients to confirm a suspected leak or abscess may prove unreliable because of their large size. Physiologic reserve is limited in this patient population so that any delay in treating a significant complication profoundly reduces a patient's ability to recover. The key to good bariatric surgical outcomes is having a high index

E-mail address: edward.livingston@utsouthwestern.edu

doi:10.1016/j.suc.2005.04.007
surgical.theclinics.com

of suspicion when patients are not progressing as expected following bariatric procedures and to reoperate on them early. It is a much better policy to explore patients on an empirical basis as soon as it is evident that the patient has the potential for a major complication rather than to wait until laboratory or imaging tests confirm the diagnosis.

Prevention

The best approach for complication management is to avoid them all together. Although there is no consensus on what clinical features contra-indicate bariatric surgery, certain features do predict surgical risk. The two most consistent features among studies investigating this issue are male gender and body size [3,8–10]. The two may be related, because men tend to be larger than women and have a propensity to accumulate fat in the abdominal compartment. Being that this fat distribution is prominent in the operative field for bariatric procedures, it increases their technical difficulty. Although there is no literature to support the practice [11], many surgeons require that large, high-risk male patients undergo some degree of preoperative weight loss. Abdominal visceral fat is one of the first compartments to lose fat. Small amounts of weight loss result in substantial reductions in visceral fat with a marked improvement in the ease of any subsequent bariatric procedure. Preoperative weight loss also establishes a patient's ability to comply with postoperative dietary regimens and may serve as a predictor for long-term success for the operation.

Age has variably been reported as a significant risk factor for complications [8]. Although older patients may be subject to higher complication rates or greater mortality when complications do occur, several series have shown that bariatric surgical procedures can be performed safely in older individuals [12–14].

Although a few series report favorable outcomes for very sick patients, those with major obesity-related complications such as oxygen-dependent hypoxia, wheelchair-bound state, pulmonary hypertension refractory to treatment, or severe congestive heart failure most likely present an excessive risk for surgery. There are series demonstrating that these patients may undergo operations with reasonable results. However, patients with this magnitude of disease do not respond very well to weight loss given that their previously physiologic defects become structural. The poor response of these disorders to weight loss places them at an unfavorable risk/benefit ratio for weight loss surgery.

Most intriguing is the relative absence of cardiovascular complications from weight loss procedures. Metabolic syndrome frequently accompanies obesity and is the underlying cause for atherosclerotic cardiovascular disease. Although patients undergoing weight loss operations tend to be relatively young, it is reasonable to assume that given the obesity–metabolic syndrome–atherosclerotic disease relationship, there would be a relatively high incidence of cardiovascular disease–related complications. In fact, these are rarely observed [1,15]. An autopsy study of patients that died following bariatric procedures found that atherosclerosis was rarely observed [16]. This coupled with the fact that many obese patients are too large to undergo preoperative cardiac testing procedures or intervention suggests that extensive preoperative cardiac evaluation is unlikely to be productive.

Specific complications

Leaks

Leaks from anastomoses or staple lines are the most feared complications. They are manifested by tachycardia and, variably, by signs of sepsis. Diagnosis of these complications can be challenging [15]. Very large patients may have little abdominal pain. Fever or elevated white blood cell counts may be absent. Even when present, these latter findings may be similar to normal postoperative changes common in bariatric surgical patients. A patient presenting with significant tachycardia (a pulse exceeding 120 beats per minute) should be considered to have a leak until otherwise proven not to have one. Leaks can occur at any time from immediately following the operation until 7 to 10 days later. When untreated, sepsis will progress, with the patient rapidly developing renal and respiratory failure.

Our policy is that, if the leak cannot be definitively ruled out, the patient should undergo surgery as soon as the suspicion for a leak arises. Gastrograffin upper gastrointestinal (GI) series examinations are helpful to establish leaks at the gastrojejunostomy or upper gastric pouch staple line. However, they do not definitively rule out leaks in other locations. Leaks of the distal stomach or its staple line will not be seen with upper GI series, nor will those of the jejunal anastomoses be reliably visualized. Diagnosis of leaks in these locations depends on visualization of intra-bdominal fluid collections with CT. Because of the large size of bariatric surgical patients, upper GI or CT studies may not provide sufficiently high-quality images to establish the diagnosis of a leak. Furthermore, patients may be too large for the gantry of these imaging devices. For these reasons, the best policy is to have a very low threshold to return a patient with a suspected leak to the operating room without delay. Failure to do so is the most common cause of preventable, major long-term disability or death in bariatric surgical patients.

Reoperations for leaks entail a thorough inspection of all regions where they may occur. These are technically challenging operations. Adequate exposure is key. If needed, incisions should be extended as far as necessary to visualize the entire operative field. Laparoscopic explorations may not reveal the source of a leak and should be converted to open procedures should the source of a suspected leak not be identified and repaired. Although the most common source for leaks is the gastrojejunostomy, other areas are prone to injury during bariatric procedures. During the process of encircling the stomach, the esophagus or posterior stomach may be torn. These areas should be carefully inspected. Methylene blue may be helpful to identify the location of these injuries if injected through a nasogastric tube. Inspecting the distal gastric pouch can be facilitated by placement of a gastrostomy tube with subsequent methylene blue injection. The gastric staple lines and the jejunal anastomosis should also be thoroughly inspected for their integrity. When possible leaks should be repaired and drains placed. When the leak cannot be identified despite a complete evaluation, or the leak cannot be repaired because of tissue inflammation, the area should be patched with omentum if possible, and drains should be placed.

Caution should be exerted in managing drains, because there is a tendency to leave them in place for long periods. Even soft silastic drains have a propensity to erode into viscera. This is especially true when there are significant amounts of tissue inflammation. When drains cease putting out substantial amounts of material, they should be removed. Replacing them operatively or by way of interventional radiological techniques is preferable to having them erode into the bowel. When drainage is low and there is a question regarding the need for a drain, a contrast tubogram will demonstrate if the drain is evacuating a significant abscess cavity of leak from the GI tract. When a drain has eroded into the bowel, diagnosis can be established with a contrast study through the drain. When this occurs, the goal is to create a controlled fistula. With time, a well-developed fistulous tract will develop and the drain can be simply removed. This generally takes 3 to 6 weeks.

Not all leaks require operative management. For patients who have few clinical manifestations of the leak that proves to be small or self-contained on contrast studies, treatment with bowel rest and parental nutritional support is possible. For patients who have major leaks in the region of the upper pouch that cannot be adequately repaired at the time of reoperation, a retrograde salem sump tube can be placed across the gastrojejunal anastomoses from the Roux-Y limb [17]. This technique facilitates long-term suction where there is a large disruption without the need to compromise respiratory function as occurs when nasogastric tubes are required. This technique has the added advantage of facilitating jejunal feeding at the site where the tube was placed retrograde in the Roux-Y limb being that patients who have recovered from a major leak have prolonged delays in recovering their ability to tolerate oral foods. An algorithm for managing leaks is presented in Fig. 1.

Pulmonary embolus

The second-most feared complication following bariatric surgery is that of pulmonary embolism. Fortunately, pulmonary embolism only occurs in 1% to 2% of cases [1,6,8], although it carries a 20% to 30% mortality [18]. These can be difficult to diagnose in the postoperative bariatric surgical

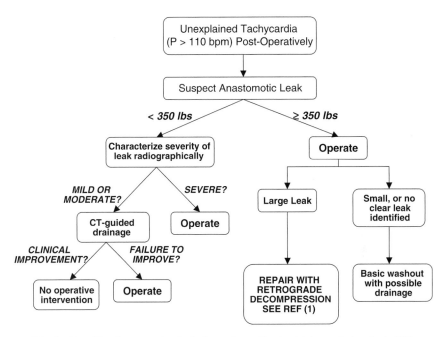

Fig. 1. Algorithm for managing leaks in postoperative bariatric surgical patients [17].

patient. Patients develop profound hypoxia. However, they will also become hypotensive with signs of sepsis indistinguishable from those observed with leaks. Consequently, when these patients present with a septic syndrome and hypoxia, both the possibility of a leak or pulmonary embolism must be simultaneously considered. They both require very different treatments so that establishing the correct diagnosis, if possible, is essential. Should the patient be small enough to fit on the CT scanning gantry, they should undergo spiral CT imaging of their chest followed by abdominal imaging. If no air or fluid collections are found in the abdomen and a pulmonary embolus is seen on the chest study, the patient should be immediately anticoagulated. In contrast, if the abdominal study demonstrates an abscess that can be percutaneously drained this should be performed. Otherwise the patient should be taken to the operating room and the abdomen explored.

The most significant dilemma arises when patients are too large to obtain any imaging studies. Under these circumstances, they should be immediately explored and, if no intrabdominal pathology is found, anticoagulation initiated. These are high-risk situations in which no good options exist and the risk of mortality is very high. For these reasons, many bariatric surgeons will not operate on individuals who are larger than the capacity of the imaging devices at the hospital where the surgery is being performed.

Prevention is always the best management strategy. Because of the high risk for thrombotic complications in this patient population, there is uniform consensus that subcutaneous anticoagulation be administered both pre- and postoperatively. However, little is known about the appropriate dosing of these agents for very large patients. In the absence of data to suggest altering dosages of these drugs in the morbidly obese, the same doses are administered as for deep venous thrombosis (DVT) prophylaxis in nonobese patients. Added protection may be conferred by placement of lower extremity compression devices during and after the operations. Often, a morbidly obese patient's legs are too large for these, so special foot pumps are used. The devices remain in place while the patient is in bed during the postoperative period.

Some surgeons recommend preoperative lower extremity duplex testing for the presence of established DVT before performing bariatric operations. When found, vena cava filters are placed to minimize the risk of postoperative pulmonary embolism. To date, evidence to support routine application of this practice is lacking.

Deep venous thrombosis

Because of their large size, morbidly obese patients are at high risk for developing DVT postoperatively following any operation. This is especially true for patients who have limited ambulation capacity before their operation. As discussed for pulmonary embolus, prevention is crucial, although the efficacy of preventive measures used for normal-sized patients has not been established for the obese [18]. DVT is manifested by the sudden onset of lower extremity edema, usually unilateral. The diagnosis may be established by duplex testing of the lower extremity venous system. Upon diagnosis, the patient should be anticoagulated with heparin and transitioned to oral warfarin therapy within the first week following development of the complication. Typically, patients are anticoagulated for 3 months following development of a DVT.

Inadequate weight loss

This complication can be the most challenging for the health care team. As many as 25% to 30% of patients undergoing bariatric surgery experience inadequate weight loss [6,19]. Patients often have unrealistic goals for themselves in terms of the degree of weight loss expected. Frequently, they seek to attain final body weights that are far less than what is achievable. Ideal body weight-for-height tables are ubiquitous, and patients will often believe that they should weigh what these tables indicate. This is rarely possible for individuals who were large enough to qualify for bariatric surgery. On average, the final weight loss is one third the initial total body weight [20]. Extensive preoperative counseling is essential regarding realistic health and weight loss goals for bariatric surgery patients.

Patients will rapidly lose weight for the first 3 months following surgery. From months 3 through 12, weight loss will be much slower but will be continuous until a plateau is reached. It is common for patients to become anxious regarding the slowed weight loss, especially as they acclimate to the operation and have less inhibition of their eating habits than was initially experienced following their procedure. Commonly, patients will express concern that the operation is no longer working. Contrast upper GI examination is appropriate to ensure the integrity of the gastric reconstruction. Once technical factors have been ruled out, patients should be referred for dietary counseling with the intent to reinforce for the patient that the operations are an adjunct to an overall dietary plan and will not result in adequate weight loss in the absence of a conscious effort at dietary control by the patient.

Many patients will experience gradual weight regain 2 to 3 years after their surgery. Once again, technical failure of the operation must be excluded, and if the surgery is found to be intact the patient is referred for dietary counseling. Operative approaches to technical failures vary depending on what the initial operation was. Vertical band gastroplasties fail in several important ways. Obstruction at the pouch outlet may result in gastroesophageal reflux disease–like symptoms, vomiting, excessive weight loss, or intractable vomiting. If the contrast upper GI series reveals an intact staple line, the pouch outlet can be resected and a Roux-Y limb of jejunum brought up as a gastric bypass to the residual pouch. Under the circumstance of an obstructed gastroplasty with an intact staple line, there is no need to revise the pouch, and attempts to do so will expose the patient to unnecessary risk for surgical complications.

Patients that have had banded gastroplasty followed by weight regain and staple line dehiscence should also be converted to a gastric bypass [21]. This operation is more extensive that that for those with obstructed pouch outlets and an intact staple line. Under these circumstances, the pouch should be dissected out and the stomach divided or re-stapled at the level of the previous staple line. A Roux-Y jejunal limb is brought to the resultant pouch creating a gastric bypass.

Patients that have regained weight with a gastric bypass that proves to be intact on contrast studies should not be offered further surgical therapy. Invariably these individuals are not compliant with dietary therapy and will fail any attempted revisional weight loss operation. This is especially true for the patient that proves to have a dilated pouch or stoma and attributes these findings to their weight gain. Reoperations to reduce the size of the pouch or stoma are technically complex and have a high complication rate. There has been extensive experience with attempts at inducing further weight loss by revising the pouch. In general, these revisions are not effective [22]. However, if the regained weight is associated with a staple line dehiscence, it is worthwhile repairing it by dividing the stomach. Under these circumstances there is a clear mechanical failure that is amenable to repair. As a rule of thumb, reoperative bariatric surgery should be kept as simple as possible. Thus, the Roux limb should not be revised unless absolutely necessary, and the staple line should be repaired only when dehiscence is clearly the reason a patient has regained weight.

Most inadvisable is the creation of a malabsorbtive limb when a conventional Roux-Y is intact. Patients with intact Roux-Y's that regain weight generally are not compliant with postoperative dietary management. Conversion of these patients to a more malabsorptive procedure is associated with substantial risk. These patients have a propensity to develop severe malabsorption followed by malnutrition. When this occurs, patients require parental nutrition until they can be restored to a normal, nutritive state. This may take several months of therapy. Once restored, these patients require reoperation with advancement of the jejunojejunostomy to a more proximal position. Another frequent complication observed in patients that have had a Roux procedure converted to a biliopancreatic diversion (BPD) is that of severe GI side effects typical of these latter procedures. Abdominal distension, pain, foul-smelling flatus, and diarrhea commonly result in these patients seeking medical care on a frequent basis. Symptoms are more severe for patients having BPD as a salvage procedure, because those who fail Roux-en-Y gastric bypass (RYGB) have a high propensity for disordered eating behaviors that result in severe GI side effects when a BPD is created.

Nutritional deficiencies

Malnutrition can occur after any weight loss procedure. Patients must be advised to have lifetime follow-up with an primary care provider and dietician. Protein-calorie malnutrition can occur. Peripheral neuropathy secondary to vitamin deficiency is surprisingly common. In a series of 435 patients undergoing bariatric procedures, 16% developed peripheral neuropathy [23]. This can be avoided by carefully monitoring a patient's postoperative diet and serum nutritional measurements. Oral vitamin supplementation can effectively avoid the development of folate deficiency [24,25] as well as iron and other vitamin and mineral deficiencies. Most gastric bypass surgeons recommend periodic systemic administration of vitamin B_{12}, because this substance's oral absorption is unreliable after these operations.

Fascial dehiscence, hernia formation, and wound infection

Fascial dehiscence occurs in approximately 1% of open bariatric cases [15,18]. The very large size of these patients coupled with some element of malnutrition postoperatively contributes to incomplete healing of fascial closures. There have been two randomized trials demonstrating that running closures are as effective as interrupted ones for obese patients undergoing bariatric procedures [26,27]. For very large patients, dehiscence risk may be minimized by placement of retention sutures to minimize the extreme amount of tension on the midline sutures that is present in the extremely obese [18].

Diagnosis of a dehiscence can be made by palpation of the fascial edges in a wound that has been opened because of an apparent infection. Small dehiscences can be managed expectantly; however, large ones should be repaired in the operating room. When a dehiscence occurs, consideration should be given to the prospect of a concomitant leak. If there is a suspicion for a leak, an upper GI examination should be obtained before reoperating on the patient if possible. If the study cannot be obtained and a leak is suspected exploration of the gastric and intestinal reconstructions should be performed at re-exploration. In most cases, the fascia cannot be reapproximated when a dehiscence has occurred. Mesh can be attached to the fascia, leaving a hernial defect. Aside from avoiding tension of the closure, leaving the abdomen open avoids abdominal compartment syndrome should there be significant intraperitoneal edema. Under these circumstances the mesh material may become infected. A greater risk is the mesh becoming attached to underlying exposed bowel that may not be covered by omentum. The author's preference is to suture Gortex to the fascia with no attempt to approximate the dehisced fascia. Several weeks after the mesh placement, it is removed. Under these circumstances, bowel adhesions will prevent evisceration, and a thick bed of granulation tissue will have formed underneath the mesh. The granulation tissue will prevent injury of otherwise exposed bowel and facilitate healing by secondary intention or skin grafting.

Incisional hernias occur in 10% to 20% of gastric bypass wounds [18,27,28]. Although avoidance of this complication is often cited as a reason to prefer the laparoscopic approach to gastric bypass, the complication is usually well tolerated. One of the most significant complaints obesity surgery patients have following weight loss is the pain and discomfort associated with loose hanging skin that is invariably present in the lower abdominal wall. Insurance companies rarely cover lipectomy procedures. However, when an incisional hernia occurs, the lipectomy can be performed concurrent to the hernia repair.

The single greatest advantage of laparoscopic approaches to Bariatric procedures is the substantial reduction in wound complications observed with laparoscopic procedures. Seromas occur in as many as 40% of open gastric bypass wounds [15]. Draining seromas is associated with little morbidity. However, when they are not adequately addressed, they evolve into wound infections [6,18]. Wound infections are treated by opening the wound and allowing it to heal by secondary intention. Antibiotics are only necessary if cellulitis surrounds the infected wound.

Marginal ulceration

The true incidence of these lesions is not well defined. They are estimated to occur in 3% to 10% of cases [18,29]. These ulcers can develop from anastomotic ischemia or excessive acid bathing the jejunal limb. Typically, the ulcer is on the jejunal side of a gastrojejunostomy and is very difficult to treat. Pain or bleeding are frequent manifestations of these lesions. Bleeding can be severe, necessitating transfusions or emergent exploration. If the pouch was made too large, it may contain a substantial amount of parietal cell mass resulting in significant acidity in the otherwise acid-free pouch environment. Staple line dehiscence results in acid traversing the incomplete staple line into the proximal gastric pouch, potentially causing marginal ulcers. Upper GI radiography will diagnose these sources of marginal ulcers. Initial treatment for marginal ulceration is done by way of administration of proton pump inhibitors. The ulcers rarely completely resolve, but medical treatment can be effective in treating hemorrhagic complications or pain. When medical treatment fails, surgery is required, with resection of the ulcer and revision of the pouch or staple line if they prove to be the underlying cause for the ulcer.

Staple line disruption

Staple line dehiscence was common with banded gastroplasties [30]. This complication, coupled with a high rate of pouch outlet obstruction or band erosion, resulted in a 35% reoperation rate for these procedures [31]. In contrast, staple line disruption with consequent weight gain is unusual following RYGB, occurring in 2% to 10% of cases [19,32]. Some have advocated dividing the stomach rather than stapling in continuity to avoid this complication. However, the risk is to develop a clinically significant leak rather than a benign gastogastric fistula, as occurs when a staple line breaks down when in-continuity stapling is employed. A prospective trial of these techniques revealed that gastrogastric fistulas were common even with divided gastric bypass, leading the authors to abandon the technique and staple in-continuity [32].

Bowel obstruction

Because few bariatric surgery series have complete, long-term follow-up, the true incidence of bowel obstruction is not known. The incidence has been reported at 2% to 3% [18] but is probably higher. Tracking of bariatric surgery patients through the California health care system for 3 years demonstrated that hospital use increased from 9% to 18% per year after these operations, with the most frequent diagnosis for admission being related to obstruction phenomena (Ko, personnel communication). Most patients can be treated with bowel rest and do not require reoperation.

Respiratory complications

Analysis of large population-based databases have consistently found respiratory disorders to be the most frequent complications of bariatric procedures [1,33]. Despite this, single institution reports almost never observe these complications [8,15]. The reason for this discrepancy is unknown, but it may reflect differences in postoperative management patterns in community hospitals, which dominate administrative databases or academic medical centers, from which most published outcome reports are derived. Extensive use of continuous positive airway pressure (CPAP) for bariatric surgery patients has been reported from a few centers [15,34] and could potentially account for the difference. CPAP assists in expanding collapsed alveoli, reducing the risk of postoperative atelectasis and pneumonia. Similarly, it has been demonstrated that nasogastric tubes are not necessary after bariatric procedures [35]. The presence of nasogastric tubes sharply reduces a patient's ability to take deep breaths and use CPAP devices. Lack of nasogastric tube use and liberal use of CPAP may account for the low rates of postoperative respiratory complications reported from a few academic medical centers.

Gallbladder disease

It is well known that gallstones form with rapid weight loss. Gallstones develop after bariatric surgery in 3% to 30% of cases [18,36]. What is not well understood is how often the de novo development of cholelithiasis after bariatric surgery results in symptomatic biliary tract disease. Postoperative administration of ursodiol following gastric bypass is highly effective in reducing gallstone formation [37]. Whereas most surgeons agree that cholecystectomy is indicated when cholelithiasis is identified during bariatric procedures, there is less agreement regarding the need for prophylactic cholecystectomy when no gallstones are identified. Cholecystectomy adds little to the overall morbidity of weight loss procedures [1]; nevertheless, because the incidence of symptomatic gallbladder disease after bariatric surgery appears to be low, most surgeons do not routinely remove the gallbladder [15].

Portal vein injury

This unusual complication can occur with bariatric procedures. We are aware of three cases in which this occurred, ultimately requiring liver transplantation. In each case, the patient died after transplantation. Although complications have been attributed to surgeon inexperience [38] in all of these cases, the operations were performed by highly experienced bariatric surgeons. Each of the three surgeons had performed at least 250 gastric bypass operations. Analysis of the complications revealed that the gastric anatomy was distorted by intraperitoneal and retroperitoneal fat deposits. In one case, the porta was lying directly anterior to the esophagus secondary to an extreme amount of retroperitoneal fat and scarring from a prior cholecystectomy. These cases highlight that experienced surgeons can be mislead by their comfort level with the operation. Even experienced surgeons should carefully assess all anatomic features of the upper quadrants before stapling the stomach, particularly noting the anatomic relationships between the porta, stomach, and esophagus.

Procedure-specific complications

Jejunoileal bypass

Although this operation was abandoned years ago, many patients underwent them and still have intact jejunoileal (JI) bypasses. They present in the modern era with a variety of complications. Patients who have had these procedures develop nephrolithiasis, hepatic failure, and cholelithiasis. They may require antimotility drugs and potassium supplementation because of chronic diarrhea. Significant nutrient malabsorption is common, frequently leading to clinical malnutrition. Despite significant malnutrition in JI patients, weight loss is less than that observed with gastric bypass [39]. Among the most pressing complications for JI bypasses were a host of vitamin and nutritional deficiencies. The presence of JI bypass was one of the significant risk factors identified in a cohort of patients undergoing bariatric surgery that developed peripheral neuropathy [23]. Patients who have had JI bypasses develop chronic infections of the bypassed limb. Excessive amounts of circulating antibodies deposit in joint spaces, causing a migratory polyarthritis. Resolution of arthritis with antibiotics characterizes this entity [40–42]. Reversal of the JI bypass is recommended.

JI bypass patients develop calcium oxalate kidney stones. Calcium oxalate is water-insoluble. In the nonbypassed bowel, oxalate deriving from green leafy vegetables is normally chelated by calcium in the small bowel, rendering it incapable of absorption in the colon. When the small bowel is bypassed, oxalate is not bound by calcium in the intestines in sufficient quantities such that free oxalate is present in the colon where it can be absorbed. When the oxalate is filtered into the kidney, the high renal oxalate concentrations facilitate creation of calcium oxalate with subsequent kidney stone formation. For these reasons, JI bypass patients should be counseled to avoid foods rich in oxalates [43].

Long-term follow-up studies revealed that JI bypass patients develop cryptogenic cirrhosis; consequently, cirrhosis is usually only diagnosed when patients present with end-stage liver disease requiring transplantation [44,45]. Because of this, and because of the many other complications of JI bypass, patients who have had these operations should be advised to have them reversed. When performing these procedures, the bypassed small bowel is atrophic, making the creation of an anastomosis difficult. Therefore, it is prudent to approach reversals as a staged operation: the jejunoileal bypass should be reversed, followed by a second procedure 6 to 12 months later to create a gastric bypass.

The biliopancreatic diversion and duodenal switch operations were designed to minimize the adverse consequences of the jejunoileal bypass operation. Although these procedures do have fewer complications, protein-calorie malnutrition remains problematic [46]. There have been no clinical trials convincing enough to recommend these procedures over gastric bypass. For this reason, few surgeons have embraced these procedures, and the number of them that are performed in the United States remains low [1].

Laparoscopic banding procedures

The safety and efficacy for these procedures remains uncertain. Although there are good long-term results from Australia and Europe, those from the United States have been mixed. Complications relating to these procedures are summarized in the articles by Drs. DeMaria and Provost elsewhere in this issue.

Laparoscopic gastric bypass

Given the similarity to the open operation, laparoscopic gastric bypass procedures have a nearly identical spectrum of complications to their open counterparts. However, there are several postoperative complications that appear to be more frequent with laparoscopic procedures. Table 1 summarizes complications reported in several publications with appreciable numbers of patients. Gastrojejunal strictures and internal hernias are more

Table 1
Complications of laparoscopic gastric bypass procedures

Complication	Higa, et al [48]	Wittgrove and Clark [49]	Schauer, et al [50]	Papasavas, et al [51]	Totals
Number of patients	1040	500	275	246	2061
Leak at gastrojejunostomy	10	11	10	4	35 (1.7%)
Gastrojejunostomy stricture requiring dilation	51	NA	13	19	83 (4.0%)
Gastrojejunostomy stricture requiring revision	1	NA	0	3	4 (0.2%)
GI bleeding requiring surgery or transfusion	6	4	6	5	21 (1.0%)
Internal hernia	26	NA	2	3	31 (1.5%)
Jejunojejunostomy obstruction	0	NA	2	3	5 (0.2%)
Stenosis at mesocolon	9	NA	0	3	12 (0.6%)
Symptomatic cholelithiasis	15	NA	4	7	26 (1.3%)
Death	5	0	1	3	9 (0.4%)

Abbreviation: NA, not available.

frequent in laparoscopic operations. Use of end-to-end anastomosis (EEA) stapling devices potentially renders the gastrojejunostomy more prone to stricture development. With the laparoscopic approach, the Roux limb is approximated to the gastric pouch without the benefit of tactile sensation. Consequently, the Roux limb is at risk for greater amounts of tension than is likely with open operations. Given that EEA staplers are frequently used in both open and laparoscopic gastric bypass operations, yet the laparoscopic procedure has a greater gastrojejunal stricture rate, creation of the Roux limb under tension is the most likely cause for this phenomenon. Creation of the gastrojejunal anastomosis with a linear stapler or hand sewing it have been proposed as alternatives to reduce stricture rates. When strictures do occur, they are easily dilated endoscopically [15].

Internal hernias are fairly common following laparoscopic gastric bypass and are rarely observed with the open procedure. Laparoscopic operations result in fewer intra-abdominal adhesions; consequently, there is less fixation of the limb and adjacent small intestine to other structures. Small bowel can easily pass in between the Roux limb and transverse mesocolon, a space known as *Peterson's defect*. With open procedures, adhesions form in this area, reducing the likelihood for internal herniation. Meticulous closure of Peterson's defect is recommended to reduce the chances of this complication; however, even with closure, internal herniation occurs relatively frequently with laparoscopic gastric bypass [47].

Deep venous thrombosis and pulmonary embolus risk are a function of patient size and were also thought to be higher in laparoscopic operations. Theoretically, reduced venous outflow from the lower extremities caused by intraoperative pneumoperitoneum increases the risk for these complications. Thus one of the concerns early in the development of laparoscopic bariatric procedures was that these risk factors would be additive resulting in a high DVT/pulmonary embolus complication rate. This has not born out, and the rate at which these complications occur appears to be similar for that observed with open gastric bypass procedures.

References

[1] Livingston EH. Procedure, incidence and complication rates of bariatric surgery in the United States. Am J Surg 2004;188:105–10.
[2] Pope GD, Birkmeyer JD, Finlayson SR. National trends in utilization and in-hospital outcomes of bariatric surgery. J Gastrointest Surg 2002;6:855–61.
[3] Nguyen NT, Paya M, Stevens CM, et al. The relationship between hospital volume and outcome in bariatric surgery at academic medical centers. Ann Surg 2004;240:586–93.
[4] Peltier G, Hermreck AS, Moffat RE, et al. Complications following gastric bypass procedures for morbid obesity. Surgery 1979;86:648–54.
[5] Balsiger BM, Kennedy FP, Abu-Lebdeh HS, et al. Prospective evaluation of Roux-en-Y gastric bypass as primary operation for medically complicated obesity. Mayo Clin Proc 2000;75:673–80.

[6] Yale CE. Gastric surgery for morbid obesity. Complications and long-term weight control. Arch Surg 1989;124:941–6.

[7] Buckwalter JA, Herbst CA Jr. Leaks occurring after gastric bariatric operations. Surgery 1988;103:156–60.

[8] Livingston EH, Huerta S, Arthur D, et al. Male gender is a predictor of morbidity and age a predictor of mortality for patients undergoing gastric bypass surgery. Ann Surg 2002;236: 576–82.

[9] Fernandez AZ Jr, DeMaria EJ, Tichansky DS, et al. Multivariate analysis of risk factors for death following gastric bypass for treatment of morbid obesity. Ann Surg 2004;239:698–702.

[10] Mason EE, Renquist KEJS. Perioperative risks and safety of surgery for severe obesity. Am J Clin Nutr 1992;55:573S–6S.

[11] Review of weight loss prior to bariatric surgery. California Department of Managed Health Care. Available at: http://www.dmhc.ca.gov/boards/cap/BariatricREV.pdf. Accessed June 25, 2005.

[12] Macgregor AM, Rand CS. Gastric surgery in morbid obesity: outcome in patients aged 55 and older. Arch Surg 1993;128:1153–7.

[13] Printen KJ, Mason EE. Gastric bypass for morbid obesity in patients more than fifty years of age. Surg Gynecol Obstet 1977;144:192–4.

[14] Papasavas PK, Gagne DJ, Kelly J, et al. Laparoscopic Roux-En-Y gastric bypass is a safe and effective operation for the treatment of morbid obesity in patients older than 55 years. Obes Surg 2004;14:1056–61.

[15] Gorecki P, Wise L, Brolin RE, et al. Complications of combined gastric restrictive and malabsorptive procedures: part 1. Curr Surg 2003;60:138–44.

[16] Melinek J, Livingston E, Cortina G, et al. Autopsy findings following gastric bypass surgery for morbid obesity. Arch Pathol Lab Med 2002;126:1091–5.

[17] Arteaga JR, Huerta S, Livingston EH. Management of gastrojejunal anastomotic leaks after Roux-en-Y gastric bypass. Am Surg 2002;68:1061–5.

[18] Brolin RE. Complications of surgery for severe obesity. Problems in general surgery 2000;17: 55–61.

[19] Sugerman HJ, Kellum JM, Engle KM, et al. Gastric bypass for treating severe obesity. Am J Clin Nutr 1992;55:560S–6S.

[20] Livingston EH, Sebastian JL, Huerta S, et al. Biexponential model for predicting weight loss after gastric surgery for obesity. J Surg Res 2001;101:216–24.

[21] Sugerman HJ, Kellum JM Jr, DeMaria EJ, et al. Conversion of failed or complicated vertical banded gastroplasty to gastric bypass in morbid obesity. Am J Surg 1996;171:263–9.

[22] Schwartz RW, Strodel WE, Simpson WS, et al. Gastric bypass revision: lessons learned from 920 cases. Surgery 1988;104:806–12.

[23] Thaisetthawatkul P, Collazo-Clavell ML, Sarr MG, et al. A controlled study of peripheral neuropathy after bariatric surgery. Neurology 2004;63:1462–70.

[24] Brolin RE, Gorman JH, Gorman RC, et al. Are vitamin B-12 and folate deficiency clinically important after Roux en-Y gastric bypass? J Gastrointest Surg 1998;2:436–42.

[25] Mallory GN, Macgregor AMC. Folate status following gastric bypass surgery (the great folate mystery). Obes Surg 1991;1:69–72.

[26] McNeil PM, Sugerman HJ. Continuous absorbable vs interrupted nonabsorbable fascial closure. A prospective, randomized comparison. Arch Surg 1986;121:821–3.

[27] Brolin RE. Prospective, randomized evaluation of midline fascial closure in gastric bariatric operations. Am J Surg 1996;172(4):328–31.

[28] Sugerman HJ, Kellum JM, Reines HD, et al. Greater risk of incisional hernia with morbidly obese than steriod-dependent patients and low recurrence with prefascial polypropylene mesh. Am J Surg 1996;171:80–4.

[29] Sapla JA, Wood MH, Sapala MA, et al. Marginal ulcer after gastric bypass: a prospective 3-year study of 173 patients. Obes Surg 1998;8:505–16.

[30] MacLean LD, Rhode BM, Forse RA. Late results of vertical banded gastroplasty for morbid and super obesity. Surgery 1990;107:20–7.

[31] Livingston EH. Obesity and its surgical management. Am J Surg 2002;184:103–13.

[32] Cucchi SG, Pories WJ, MacDonald KG, et al. Gastrogastric fistulas. A complication of divided gastric surgery. Ann Surg 1995;221:387–91.

[33] Liu JH, Zingmond D, Etzioni DA, et al. Characterizing the performance and outcomes of obesity surgery in California. Am Surg 2003;69:823–8.

[34] Huerta S, DeShields S, Shpiner R, et al. Safety and efficacy of postoperative continuous positive airway pressure to prevent pulmonary complications after Roux-en-Y gastric bypass. J Gastrointest Surg 2002;6:354–8.

[35] Huerta S, Arteaga JR, Sawicki MP, et al. Assessment of routine elimination of postoperative nasogastric decompression after Roux-en-Y gastric bypass. Surgery 2002;132:844–8.

[36] Amaral JF, Thompson WR. Gallbladder-disease in the morbidly obese. Am J Surg 1985;149: 551–7.

[37] Sugerman HJ, Brewer WH, Shiffman ML, et al. Ursodiol acid prevents gallstone formation following gastric bypass induced rapid weight loss: a multicenter placebo controlled, randomized double-blind prospective trial. Am J Surg 1994;169:91–6.

[38] Flum DR, Dellinger EP. Impact of gastric bypass operation on survival: a population-based analysis. J Am Coll Surg 2004;199:543–51.

[39] Griffen WO Jr, Young VL, Stevenson CC. A prospective comparison of gastric and jejunoileal bypass procedures for morbid obesity. Ann Surg 1977;186:500–9.

[40] Corrodi P, Wideman PA, Sutter VL, et al. Bacterial flora of the small bowel before and after bypass procedure for morbid obesity. J Infect Dis 1978;137:1–6.

[41] Drenick EJ, Ament ME, Finegold SM, et al. Bypass enteropathy. Intestinal and systemic manifestations following small-bowel bypass. JAMA 1976;236:269–72.

[42] Passaro E Jr, Drenick E, Wilson SE. Bypass enteritis. A new complication of jejunoileal bypass for obesity. Am J Surg 1976;131:169–74.

[43] Hassan I, Juncos LA, Milliner DS, et al. Chronic renal failure secondary to oxalate nephropathy: a preventable complication after jejunoileal bypass. Mayo Clin Proc 2001;76: 758–60.

[44] Lowell JA, Shenoy S, Ghalib R, et al. Liver transplantation after jejunoileal bypass for morbid obesity. J Am Coll Surg 1997;185:123–7.

[45] Markowitz JS, Seu P, Goss JA, et al. Liver transplantation for decompensated cirrhosis after jejunoileal bypass: a strategy for management. Transplantation 1998;65:570–2.

[46] Picard M, Frederic SH, Stefane L, et al. Complications of combined gastric restrictive and malabsorptive procedures: part 2. Curr Surg 2003;60:274–9.

[47] Higa KD, Ho T, Boone KB. Internal hernias after laparoscopic Roux-en-Y gastric bypass: incidence, treatment and prevention. Obes Surg 2003;13:350–4.

[48] Higa KD, Boone KB, Ho T, et al. Laparoscopic Roux-en-Y gastric bypass for morbid obesity: technique and preliminary results of our first 400 patients. Arch Surg 2000;135: 1029–33.

[49] Wittgrove AC, Clark GW. Laparoscopic gastric bypass, Roux-en-Y- 500 patients: technique and results, with 3–60 month follow-up. Obes Surg 2000;10:233–9.

[50] Schauer PR, Ikramuddin S, Gourash W, et al. Outcomes after laparoscopic Roux-en-Y gastric bypass for morbid obesity. Ann Surg 2000;232:515–29.

[51] Papasavas PK, Caushaj PF, McCormick JT, et al. Laparoscopic management of complications following laparoscopic Roux-en-Y gastric bypass for morbid obesity. Surg Endosc 2003;17:610–4.

ELSEVIER
SAUNDERS

Surg Clin N Am 85 (2005) 869–874

SURGICAL
CLINICS OF
NORTH AMERICA

Index

Note: Page numbers of article titles are in **boldface** type.

Changing Your Address?

Make sure your subscription changes too! When you notify us of your new address, you can help make our job easier by including an exact copy of your Clinics label number with your old address (see illustration below.) This number identifies you to our computer system and will speed the processing of your address change. Please be sure this label number accompanies your old address and your corrected address—you can send an old Clinics label with your number on it or just copy it exactly and send it to the address listed below.

We appreciate your help in our attempt to give you continuous coverage. Thank you.

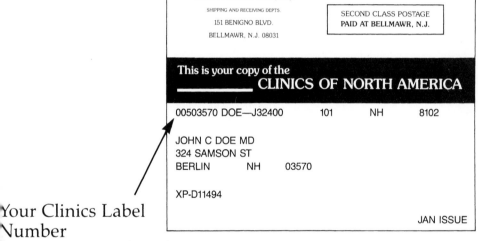

W. B. Saunders Company

SHIPPING AND RECEIVING DEPTS.
151 BENIGNO BLVD.
BELLMAWR, N.J. 08031

SECOND CLASS POSTAGE
PAID AT BELLMAWR, N.J.

This is your copy of the
_____ **CLINICS OF NORTH AMERICA**

00503570 DOE—J32400   101   NH   8102

JOHN C DOE MD
324 SAMSON ST
BERLIN   NH   03570

XP-D11494

JAN ISSUE

Your Clinics Label Number
Copy it exactly or send your label along with your address to:
W.B. Saunders Company, Customer Service
Orlando, FL 32887-4800
Call Toll Free 1-800-654-2452

Please allow four to six weeks for delivery of new subscriptions and for processing address changes.